Cultivating a Body of Nectar

Kriya Yoga and Tantric Foundations

CULTIVATING A BODY OF NECTAR

KRIYA YOGA AND TANTRIC FOUNDATIONS

Virochana Khalsa

Books of Light Publishing

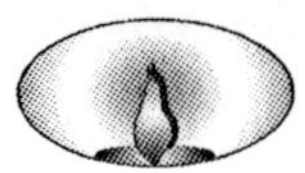

Books of Light Publishing
PO Box 576
Crestone, CO 81131 USA
mvk@silverearth.com

Printed in the Unites States of America
Palatino 10.5/14 60# paper 288 pages

ISBN 1-929952-04-X *paperback*

Note: This book was previously to be titled:
Creating an Eternal Body, Part One: Kriyas and Preliminary Practices.

CONTENTS

Dedication

This book is dedicated to the Eternal Masters.
In dedicating the book in this way, it automatically becomes available for the benefit of all people.

. . . . .

To say all the ways I am grateful for and to Whitecloud, my Beloved TwinRay, would require more pages than this book has. Simply, in my eyes and heart she is the eloquence of Love and Wisdom through clarity.

Thanks

Thanks to Shivayas for his help.

Preface

Presented here are methods to become more grounded, present, connected and clear, thereby creating a foundation in which to better apply ourselves on our spiritual journey. For those who simply want to use these practices solely for better health, more clarity and enjoyment that is fine.

For those who want to go further a few techniques are presented to begin creating the inner temple and its body of nectar, without which the higher tantras, i.e., ascension practices, have no foothold. To this aim a detailed presentation of our chakras, channels, energy and essences is given with insights gained through years of practice.

Ascension is a subject that has received a lot of press, most of it with little in-depth understanding. While the term *Ascension* was brought into use by western mystics, it is an accomplishment that has been worked for and realized by thousands over the millennia in many different lands. Ascension is not about enlightenment, which is its continual starting point, rather about the radiance of that enlightenment into an eternal body that can display itself beyond the unconscious wheel of birth and death.

In addressing such a mountainous subject as Ascension, where do we start? As with everything else, precede one step at a time and just keep walking forward. If an area seems too advanced right now, go ahead and look into it anyway, while continuing what is right for you at this time. You are planting seeds to flower in your time. An example is the very subtle understanding of emptiness[1].

If it is not time yet to embrace this depth of reality at least expose your self to it. Then when it naturally begins to reveal itself, you will be in a much better place to understand it (and enter the bliss within it). The expanding of perspective helps in every walk of life. When the four-minute mile was broken, the expansion of perspective helped many more to do it. When a culture excels in an area, this perspective naturally accelerates all those who desire to explore this area.

By exposing your self to the inner workings of Ascension it moves from an area of mystery, religion and fantasy to the realms of application, nature and possibility. By applying yourself in this science, the beautiful artwork of your soul is laid bare, forever creating and changing through the power of your spirit; thus our spirit is known.

Few will take these teachings to their fullness in one lifetime, but many can gain enough to create a momentum that their soul will carry forwards. So even a little bit of practice is of great value.

1 For those of a scientific mind, I recently read that according to a prominent physics theory, there is enough potential energy within one cubic centimeter of a vacuum to boil all the water in all the oceans of our world, if only someone could figure out how to tap into it.

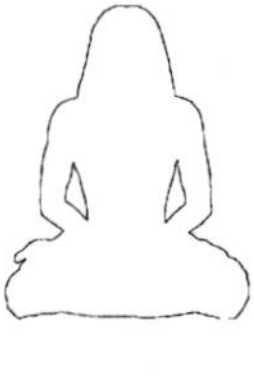

1

Overview

This chapter overviews what this series of books are about, while introducing some key concepts, terms, and understanding. It is recommended that you read this chapter several times.

Cultivating a Body of Nectar

Without bliss, the path is dry and filled with pursuits and doubts of the mind. Without bliss, experience comes and goes; yet nothing much changes. Bliss is timeless, it reveals our true nature, it consumes and creates, bliss is the fuel for the spiritual path.

A few times in new classes, I have asked ***"how many here have experienced real, mind blowing, full of light, consuming bliss through their practice."*** These are classes with people who have been meditating or doing the "spiritual path" for quite a few years. To my surprise, each time only a few people raised their hands, and often with some deliberation at that.

Spirituality, the art of knowing our spirit, is a very blissful affair. Nectar is our essence that makes spirit knowable in form and creating a body of nectar is a science that any of us can do. In this book, methods are given to create enough clarity and vitality to cultivate the nectars of bliss.

Bliss consumes dogma, religion, prejudices, and fantasies. It lifts us naked and in silent depth it implodes and explodes. Bliss can hold the straightest face, walk the cleanest line, be the most grounded and make the most sense; in happiness, tranquility, compassion, even sadness and anger; a blissful being, always forgetting, never forgets who they are, because it is our nature lied bare and beautiful.

This book is not about instant fixes, rather creating a foundation in which to permanently reside. A body of nectar is cultivated, not instantly made manifest through fantasy and wishing. Through this body of nectar we are fit to obtain all of who we are, for we have a body that can be it all. Let's start ...

Yogic Development and the Preliminaries

Preliminaries focus on grounding, connectivity and presence through the yogic path of self-development. Thus this is primarily a practice manual filled with priceless methods. With this foundation we can reach for the sky with our feet in spirit-nectar, which is the subject of the remaining books in this series.

Practicing techniques without integration into our everyday life only gets us so far. Besides, why not adjust our lifestyle so as to create an atmosphere of discovery and richness? Areas of relationship, emotion, sexuality, self-responsibility, motivation, morality, diet, attitude, what we do for work and environment are all a vital part of self-development. Lifestyle and character are only briefly discussed in this book. There is not so much a formula, rather an obviousness of approach and emotional richness that becomes apparent as we continue. The details are usually somewhat different for each of us and at different times in our lives.

There is a saying, "more practice, less drama, less practice more drama." The movement of energy and deepening awareness that occurs through yogic practice clears away much of the toxic and neurotic aspects of our life. In the first years of this stage of practice we are not so interested in the content of our emotions as in the radiance of our being. Then, and only then, can we really listen to what our emotions are saying to us, in perspective, and thereby use the energy of emotion as an integrated and necessary part of our clarity.

Yogic development revolves around a combination of passive and active practice. A *Kriya* is an active practice that often uses a combination of breath (subtle and physical), visualization, mantra, posture, and even dynamic movement to create and deepen a nonverbal presence that supports meditative strengthening, deepening and discovery. In short kriyas help to clear agitation, introduce us to the potential of our body and mind and make us fit enough to one-pointedly apply ourselves.

Passive practice is where we give up and surrender. It is meditating through the natural wisdom of open awareness. Passive meditation is possible when the agitation of the mind cannot pull you in a million directions, because the inner space is much more seductive, natural and vast than the quibbling and apparent force of the outer mind. There is not so much any one technique as a readiness for it. A typical example is still, silent meditation where you just sit. At first, most people will have to move through agitation, and then boredom. If you can simply remain with and inside yourself after awhile your radiance peeks through the boredom. It is inevitable, because there is nothing else going on. Your life-force is becoming one-pointed in its own natural intrinsic quality of bliss, and this bliss, when truly known, holds the outer mind in a much greater attraction than anything of the world can. If anything else is going on, you give up on it, not because you have to, but because you want to (although at first, you give up on it through faith in the practice). When you really give up, not like a depression, but in a way of letting go of anything or any one or even your own idea of self, you relax into a radiant-emptiness. It is a very open feeling – which develops a true sense of awareness where space and spatial qualities are not physical distance but a conscious quality of attunement. Without this openness it is difficult to trust that the spiritual path has more validity than the struggle. We simply give up on our intellect, grasping and pride as anything that is going to get us anywhere. This openness is the only way to move past doubt.

Kriyas will open up an inner space, which will give you a feeling of this openness and oneness of existence *(the one flavor)*. But it is transitory. Through the passive practices, you discover it independent of props. A person can do lots of kriyas and techniques, but they just become part of the wheel of endless experience until a person gives up on the wheel. When a person is willing to apply this aspect of the path, then they are truly ready. Everything else is secondary: work, happiness, everything is the scenery. Later, we reintegrate with the scenery in a very spectacular way. But, if we try to do it from an egotistical sense, it just becomes an egotistical extension.

Passive practices are not given in the beginning; rather one has to be ripe for it. You have to have had enough experience to know that there is something more. Then the active techniques get you clear enough so that you actually have the capacity to sit through boredom long enough to ground within the vastness of inner space and discover something else. A core of prana is developed that can support a fullness of awareness that is rich and effortlessly nonverbal, and within that you deepen into and relax within your true nature. A passive practice is not going for a walk, or taking a sleep. It is a very deep penetration of dissolving and then rediscovering ourselves. To really open up and let go requires a magnetic grounding inside of our bodies. To be grounded inside our bodies requires connectivity. Then we can let go from an inner core, and the effect is total. Spacing out is not a very effective passive practice. This is not about dullness or sleepiness or excitation, rather a deeper presence that we are beyond grasping. It is often the first experience of unconditioned bliss, even if only a cozy bliss. The two practices, active and passive work hand in hand.

The working together of active and passive practice opens the tantric path. Through the specifics of particular techniques and the skill of relaxing our ego, we learn how to remain within our inner core. Within this originality of ourselves, emptiness and radiance does not have to be searched after, rather it is the original and natural condition. When we go to the ocean, we do not have to imagine what water looks like, because it is the scenery, it is the environment, and in this case it is us.

Eternal Yoga[1]

The next book in this series introduces Eternal Yoga, which is a way of discovering our eternal nature. In this practice we go above the head to aid this discovery. It is here that we understand our body, soul and spirit without any doubt as to what is meant by these terms. By bringing forth a bigger expanse, we have the opportunity for much greater self-definition. In this radiant clarity we will learn how to release the contraction of our individual grasping so that we gain freedom within our truer nature. These practices form the foundation for further advancement on the spiritual journey, of which the various options are examined.

During this time, we will become aware of the Ascended Masters or accomplished Buddhas in a way that is not separate from us. Non-dualism becomes more than just a word as "we get there by being there." The whole spiritual path starts to warm-up in a very special way and we begin to realize that enlightenment, ascension and the body of light are all actual possibilities.

Through the activations of Eternal Yoga, we gain the ability to see and overcome our seed karmas. Awareness within our subtle body of light is necessary to even consider a path of liberation within a lifetime or two. The Blessing Presence so developed becomes the conduit of transmission and merit that makes our continued growth possible.

Tantra

The third book in this series is about the higher tantras, whereby we birth a consciousness that is eternally awake in our true nature within, through, and as form.

Tantra is the continuum gained by grounding the perspective of our existence into an inner core that resides beyond the frozen limitations of conventional life.

Practical methods are given in the tantra book to gain awareness of and then ground within this core. As we advance, we are able to

1 Eternal yoga is a term given to us by an Ascended Master near the end of an intensive training from several ascended masters during a retreat in the Himalayas, with the instructions, "that this is what you are to teach."

use our desires, passions and characteristics as the basic energy to enlighten our natural state. It begins by sharpening the vision gained in Eternal Yoga, of making everything appear more transparent, less solid and as the outer skin of an underlying divinity. In doing so, we ignite an inner core of presence within our body and through further skillful application we create an inner temple from which our appearance radiates forth. The possibility of bringing forth an eternal body of consciousness presents itself within this development of the nectar body.

While the popular understanding in America of the word tantra is about sex, a truer understanding is development of a refined energy body. As a path, tantra starts with development of the inner temple and concerns itself with the continuum and the continuity of conscious presence. Tantric practices work with passion and blending as part of the path, and thus sexual union is an invaluable aspect, provided the ability and awareness of working with refined energy is already present.

Tantra is a path of a thousand corrections enroute. A disposition that is rigid, or one that does not understand the how and why of various practices, will not intuitively be able to make these corrections. This fluidity is impossible if a person is rigidly bound within constraints of social consciousness. Sensitivity to these thousand plus corrections requires that we listen, and it is one of the reasons that an experienced teacher is necessary. A few advanced souls can get this feedback through subtle interaction with a teacher, but most require a physical interaction.

Tantra is a path of intensity and transformation, where we intensify our passions while bringing them into the emptiness of our inner temple. The bliss within that indivisible union reveals the perfection that underlies everything. We let go while simultaneously radiating profound existence in all its varied peculiarities and plays.

The Great Perfection

The Great Perfection is in essence a path beyond technique, being the state of enlightenment. Some practitioners focus on first tasting, through transmission, the Great Perfection and then blossoming this awareness into fruition.

The great perfection is also called "dzog-chen" in the Tibetan teachings and in the west was presented in a profound, yet seldom-understood and greatly miss-represented path called the "I Am." It is very simple, direct, and at the same time an extremely advanced approach. The flavor of the Great Perfection is constantly interwoven, quite deeply so, within Eternal Yoga and the tantric journeys presented in this series of books.

Any non-dualistic approach, such as the higher tantras, must by definition of "non-dualistic" use the underlying empowerment of the Great Perfection – "we get there by being there." The Great Perfection is both the beginning and the end. Eternal Yoga enters us from the level of higher-mind into the Great Perfection understanding. How we then choose to encompass every aspect of life into our realization decides whether we embrace the skillful means of the Tantric path or continue solely within the Great Perfection path.

Both Tantra and the pure Great-Perfection paths if followed to completion have the same end result. Journeying the tantric path, because of the development of skilful means, gives an ability to benefit more people. Skilful means and transformation is used in Tantra to progressively awaken within the all-encompassing sphere of the Great Perfection. The Great Perfection approach, by itself, uses pure awareness and its inherent energy as the path itself. There is nothing to embrace, no vows to keep, nothing to transform, just pure awareness itself revealing itself. There is a 'dzog-chen saying, "The sickness of effort has been overcome."

Through maintaining awareness, within that awareness the transmission occurs which reveals the underlying elemental light-play of form and formlessness. Because the practitioner has learned to unwaveringly remain aware, this transmission of the light-play remains ever present, "lifting," "deepening" and "absorbing" ones everyday awareness into the power and presence inherent within it. In short, the eternal body is gained within and as the fluidic play of life.

It requires an infinite ability of fluidity and its one absolute dependence is in bringing forth a relationship with a master or masters whereby the transmissions may occur in consciousness.

Dream Yoga

There are two aspects of dream yoga. One is cultivating the ability to dream with clarity and lucidity. In this state we can do practice, project ourselves, gain understanding, perform service and transform the nature and content of our dreams.

A more advanced aspect of dream yoga is not about dreams at all, rather absorbing our pranas within our central core and maintaining radiant primal consciousness while we sleep. This is an aspect of tantric practice.

Of course we all, regardless of spiritual practice or not, at times have pertinent and lucid dreams. However dream yoga is experiencing this consistently. Practices to facilitate dream awareness and radiant awareness while asleep will be given in a later book in this series.

Dream yoga is an incredible valuable part of practice. Success in this is a reflection of our daytime practice. Trying to gain mastery in this area without a strong daytime practice is extremely difficult if not impossible. However in times of intense practice, such as during a retreat, dream clarity and remaining awake within our core while asleep often occurs spontaneously and as a kind of after effect - a continuation of our daytime practice.

Motivation

Within our growth through these methods is a concurrent refinement of our motivation, which may also be called an opening of our heart. As we clean our own house, the ambition to achieve greater enlightened activity and presence changes from a self-centered activity to altruistic love and compassion. Far from the mushy heart, this is tremendous clarity born of and blended with wisdom beyond a conventional mind-set. The desire to benefit all beings as the cause of our enlightenment and as a radiance that breaks through our contraction is simply reflective of the deeper radiant nature of reality. The ascended body is nothing other than the "body of the one." The growing change of motivation within us is a clear sign as to our readiness to embrace the next stages.

Tantra blossoms into a free flowing blessing power through a heart-centered, good-natured, yet not naïve attitude.

The tantric path is to be or to become a Blessing Presence.

Any other motivation plays havoc, because it is afraid of loosing something called self.

It is my observation that until a person is comfortable and clear in regards to relationship, sexuality and intimacy they are not yet ready for the tantric path. Being able to work with ones energy in a conscious, empowered and surrendered way (required in relationship) is part of this path.

A Teacher

In the more common spiritual paths, such as religion, the outer yogas, self-reflection, purification, etc., it is not absolutely necessary to have a teacher. However as the tantric path is entered fully, a teacher or teachers are necessary for reasons of transmission and because of how quickly difficult areas of the psyche are entered into. The relationship with a teacher is very sacred. Only those people who live in sacredness can understand this relationship. The tantric path requires divine intimacy, respect and wisdom with a teacher to facilitate the necessary ongoing transmission.

In the oneness of life we learn something by first experiencing a feeling or sense of it and then embodying that feeling under our own image so that it becomes a natural part of our being. This is a primary function of transmission, i.e., the direct sharing of divine experience.

Without transmission there is no real clear understanding of where we are going. It is all just words. There are many scriptural accounts of how students have undergone years or decades of service, preparation and growth to enter into a space where transmission can occur, and where they are consciously aware of it. Once profound transmission is experienced, then it is only a matter of application and stabilization, for the result has already been attained on a seed level. We get there by being there. While I am talking about profound transmission, the many thousands of small transmissions, the nuances we pick up from enlightened company and communion are a vital part of the spiritual path.

A teacher on the spiritual path is someone you have given authority to. Thus this person can question you, provoke and stimulate you, and communicate to you in areas you may not otherwise allow. Obviously this requires surrender. Confusion arises in some people because they equate surrender with giving away their power or worship. However, real surrender is impossible in a framework of disempowerment or blind worship and cannot occur as long as the lower mind plays around in confusion and a toxic way. You must still do the work. Thus a real relationship with a teacher is a mature and advanced state of sensitive communion. The outer mind becomes still.

For most people tantra is about passion and blending. Emotion, feeling and passion are, as we become clear, the voltage that makes all this possible. As this happens then our feeling ability opens up an inner all pervading space, which is infinitely delicate and embracing. There is an inspiring beauty of using attachment, desire, intimacy and emotion to fuel our awakening within the natural state. Without a pure relationship with someone who understands what we are being refined into, this process will become a circus and not yield the type of fruit that allows the work to begin on the Ascended body within the space of one lifetime. **A tantric teacher will use the power of emotion to bring forth definition within the emptiness, not within a mindset fixed on social conditioning.**

Ascension

Ascension is about form and more specifically is a western term for an aspect of the higher Tantras and the Great-Perfection in which a vision is unveiled of the elemental quality of the mind. This vision extends into how we see everything, and in this, our body is transformed into a direct active expression of this elemental mind. In short, we transform our physical body into a body of light that remains active within the physical and subtle realms.

There are various levels of mastery within this light body and who can perceive its appearance. For example, there are masters who can temporarily project such a body as a penetration of their forever-existing extremely subtle body, those who effortlessly sustain it, those who can only sustain it within the consciousness of the earth and those who can sustain it anywhere in the universe.

How regular physical people perceive such a Master is a combination of a person's sensitivity, interior language, and a manipulation by the master of the visual ability of others to perceive them. For example, there are yogis whom we have had contact with that are visible to some people and not to others.

A fully developed body of light can only come about by the desire to benefit others; otherwise, because of self-absorption, it would not come about in this fullness. This body is not, in wisdom, the same as ghostly apparitions or a temporary karmic projection from a being in god-like realms.

****

This is a good place to have a break and absorb what you have read.

****

Enlightenment and the Tantras

The starting point of the higher tantras is enlightenment, which is an experience of the all-pervading space of consciousness, i.e., emptiness, and oneness, radiant with clarity and purity presenting itself as the display of form, such as yourself and all that you see. What this is saying is that there is no concrete building block of the universe other than consciousness itself. The choice of which descriptive term of enlightenment is emphasized varies according to the context of how we experienced manifestation as arising from within this basic reality.

By learning to relax into our nonverbal, alive and effortless presence as a center in which all outer manifestation and thoughts absorb into and come out of, then through that center we enter into the vastness without a center. It is a wonderful play. This frees us of our grasping nature and with this foundational experience we can apply ourselves in an enlightened perspective into further penetration and integration, i.e., the higher tantras.

Enlightenment, when stripped of mysticism and recognized is relatively easy to experience (as a sense of radiant-clarity) in moments but much more challenging to integrate with all that is in a state of continuity. Thus tantra is about the continuum and continuity of conscious. Underlying all consciousness is an energetic support. Consciousness and energy are inseparable, and on the deepest levels – consciousness creates its own supporting energy. Tantra as a science is about working with the continuum of the energy body.

When a person feels as pointless the continual circulation of unending experiences and instead desires to become established in a state of dynamic fulfillment, then the time is ripe to step off the wheel and enter the primal presence of our very being.

Tantra is a non-dual approach — in other words "you get there by being there." This most critical understanding is the source of empowerment, the ability to use transmission, and the difference between religious entanglement and spiritual freedom. Simply put you gain initial experience and keep on cultivating and refining it into the blossoming of your fullness. This is a yogic path, so nothing is outside of yourself, but you will have to surrender to that.

My initiation and development on the higher tantras, in this life, in partnership with my beloved twin-ray, occurred primarily through transmission and reflection with various subtly embodied masters. Thus I developed my own terminology and methodology to communicate the process. In this series of books I hope to bridge, to the best of my ability, my experience and terminology with some of the long-standing, true and tried tantric paths. This combination hopefully gives a freshness that the reader can interface with the already existing tantric texts and methods.

The Three Kayas of Body, Soul & Spirit

Skillful application of Tantra is dependent on becoming familiar with the qualities of body, soul and spirit. The Buddhists call the enlightened body, soul and spirit the three kayas: the *dharmakaya* (spirit), *sambhogakaya* (a very subtle body formed from the radiance of spirit) and *nirmanakaya* (physical). Because of their emphases on the enlightenment of these aspects and certain other subtleties I shall mostly use the Buddhist terms[1].

The process of gaining familiarity with the three kayas evolves from one stage to the next, but becomes particularly alive within *Eternal Yoga*.

Through consistent practice the meaning of the three kayas will become as familiar to you as your own name. Dharmakaya is our spirit, our I-Am presence as referred to in some western traditions, and in the tantras as our consciousness which radiates out from the inner-most all pervading existence of everything. It is the center of which there is no center. It is beyond and prior to our continually qualified images of soul and body. It is not something that we can reach by way of a projection, identity, or subtle vehicle but a depth of ourselves we recognize. This recognition often starts as a very subtle and quiet intuitive cognition or sense, and we use that as an anchor to help us get there by being there. It is simply clarity. A clear teacher can help us to recognize what is already within us and thus draw it into our practice.

Stabilized awareness of our formless source is entered through transmission and lots of meditative familiarity (practice). The dharmakaya as a point of empowerment is ultimately the only way we can gain the self-definition needed for ascension. Also symmetrical alignment (in our energy body) with our dharmakaya keeps us from running off-track. This alignment is the deeper understanding of purity and wisdom together. Learning how to access this point of empowerment is a teaching of Eternal Yoga. Our dharmakaya aspect is beyond soul, yet it can be seen by anyone who is awakened within it.

The sambhogakaya is a very subtle radiant image and activity that is solely created from mind-pranas. Mind-prana is energy that effortlessly and spontaneously originates out of nothingness and is the primal radiance of our mind. Out of nothingness means that this

1 In its most refined understanding, the Taoist description of *Shen* is spirit, Shen and *Chi* (energy) is soul, and Shen, Chi, and *Jieng* (sexual essence) is body. The nature of Shen is Wu Chi (emptiness), yet it very name recognizes that even the emptiness originates a Chi. From the pure level of spirit all is emptiness and its radiance (chi). In the Taoist approach, Jieng is refined into its pure origination from Chi. We refine our Chi to support a greater aliveness of Shen (our spirit), thus Chi is refined into Shen or the Dharmakaya. In this way the continuum and inseparability of life is understood. The Taoist approach has many wonderful gems (methods and understandings) to help us gain greater awareness through a practical application within our bodies, environment and energy awareness.

energy does not originate from our food, the air we breathe, outer sensory input or any form of self-contraction. The tantric path is totally entwined in the development of, activity and overseer ship by our sambhogakaya self.

Seeing within these realms and integrating that experience with our life is the only practical way of overcoming our self-created obstacles. Self-obsession, arrogance, lack of humility and indifference to others is a quick way to turn the sambhogakaya experience into another trap, one that is difficult to get out of, because one becomes a sort of prideful god with lots of power to maintain that blinded position. The mind is infinitely resourceful which can be either its liberation or bondage.

Both the dharmakaya and sambhogakaya have several different aspects of consciousness or subtle energy that makes up these spheres of activity. Each has a gateway of consciousness. For the dharmakaya I call this the gateway of purity or the emptiness. For the sambhogakaya it is the crown chakra in the head. As previously mentioned, consciousness and subtle energy are two sides of the same coin and can never be separated from each other. However a dominance of view can occur. The energy dominant view is the etheric aspect and the consciousness dominant view is the mental aspect. The etheric aspect of the sambhogakaya is the eighth realm just above the head and the mental aspect is the ninth realm further above the head. The eighth realm creates the initial structure of the chakras and principle channels of energy in the body. The ninth realm is a place of blessing presence for and inter-related with all beings, whereby we can radiate forth as a dynamic truth in all of creation.

The Nirmanakaya is our physical body and physical-dependent energy bodies (such as our dream body). When through the empowerment of our spirit, we originate the reality of our physical body from the consciousness of our soul, we have a body that is not dependent on gross relativity (i.e., food and air) and thus from this framework it is deathless. This is the process of Ascension.

Familiarity of these aspects is not enough to gain an ascended body. This requires the intimate integration of the higher tantras. In the completion stage we create an inner temple from which we experience ourselves emanating forth. This requires a lot of self-definition and a simultaneous dissolving of our identity. The feeling of this will have already been touched upon previously but now we are going all the way. The boundaries of inner and outer disappear along with dualistic consciousness.

How thoroughly this occurs is the result of what is believed possible and what is worked for within the framework of being a blessing presence for all beings. Creating an eternal body in the physical is a rare, yet possible activity that requires a consciousness in every area of life. This series of books will address the differences in approach between an eternal body in the very subtle realm of pure potential (sambhogakaya) and the physical (nirmanakaya).

Why Create an Eternal Body?

When you no longer feel the need to create an eternal body because you are afraid of dying, or because you are afraid of not existing, then you can answer this more fully for yourself.

Liberation, from the spiritual fullness of the word, requires creation of an eternal body on at least a rarefied realm of existence. How much this consciousness can penetrate, while remaining conscious, into denser realms of existence, is the degree of your ascension and the realization of your nectar body. We all have within us Buddha nature, however not all of us have actualized it. There are all sorts of possibilities. It is up to each of us what we want to actualize.

Activity is aliveness. Activity has a form. To remain alive we must remain in form. How, where and on what level we want to remain alive determines how and where we want to have the existence of a body. Passive awareness is what spiritually occurs when we become an all-pervading quality without a "specific" active vehicle. Compassion, the active flow of love, is the only force that can maintain an active body at this level of existence. To become self-absorbed in tranquil-bliss, beyond the notice of form, is nirvana. We have become the bliss quality of the universe. When others experience bliss, they are by the quality of oneness, one with us. Yet we are no longer an active principle, because we ourselves are totally absorbed as this quality. It is similar to (although more conscious than) a refreshing dreamless sleep, or to a deep tranquil, body-forgetting meditation where nothing is happening. For some this is there spiritual goal. It is deeply restful. This is the opposite of creating an active body.

Having absorbed ourselves totally in the nirvana of our tranquil bliss, evaporating almost all notice of form, eventually, some being becomes actively one with our state, and in a very attractive splendor, penetrates a sense of compassionate aliveness into our being in a defined way. Inspired by this indescribable splendor of aliveness, a desire is awoken in us to take an active role. Then we instantaneously create a subtle body (of already existing potential) and through relativity, descend into a physical embodiment to begin again. It is a cycle of compassion and absorption and is a subtle way of being bound within cause and effect, until we learn how to be both absorbed and extroverted at the same time. This is the power of Love, the seduction of Bliss and the totality of the play of Emptiness[1].

Active awareness results from playing in the world of relativity, i.e., my apparent body and your apparent body. In creating an eternal body, we never totally absorb ourselves in nirvana. Rather we have a foot in each door (in an expanded sense). An Eternal Body becomes a vehicle of great service, which in the world of oneness, is consciousness and radiance at play. The only way that such a radiance of consciousness can occur, as a continuing continuum, is through the love of all beings. This flow of love is the bliss of life.

It is possible to have developed a subtle vehicle (our soul) in a higher realm and yet remain ignorant here on earth. In this case, our enlightened self has incarnated its essence here on earth to awaken here on earth.

1 In the search for love, we develop like and dislike. In the wanting of Bliss, we become ambitious. In the illusion of self, we distract ourselves in a million ways and never rest in the effortlessness of true nature. The cure for all these afflictions is the very thing we seek, or want, yet because of distraction, we are not clear in what it is we want or seek. Thus the first step is clarity, i.e., quieting the mind and resting in clarity. Yoga has wonderful methods to achieve this. Following this is to cultivate the natural state of our budhhic nature. Prana is what keeps us awake and bliss is a radiance of prana. Thus in the wanting of prana, we check our ambition to keep it flowing in a direction from and towards the effortless wisdom of the enlightened state. It is like an energetic kid who can find a million things to do, but with right direction matures into fullness. It requires a lot of application and hard work to become effortless, but then it is much harder to remain trapped in illusion.

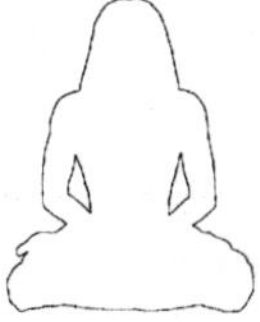

2

Lifestyle Adjustments

" Spirituality becomes alive only when everyday life becomes a divine experience"

- Whitecloud Khalsa

Healthy Environment and Right Livelihood

Whitecloud emphasizes that environment is at least fifty percent of the spiritual path. For myself, I felt that this was somewhat of an exaggeration, but over the years I am beginning to appreciate the wisdom of this outlook.

Living in a place of nature, and out of the demanding pace of the city and its occupations, supports greater clarity. Of course a neurotic city person will most likely become a neurotic rural person. But if a person can quite him or herself and attunes with nature's honesty, energy and inner reflection, then this is a tremendous support. When I lived in Los Angeles I felt that I was doing several yoga sets a day just to clear the physical and psychic pollution.

Creating an appropriate environment includes the type of work we do and the social activities we engage in. I believe that each person understands in their moments of clarity for him or herself what is best at particular times in their life. It takes courage to change and to trust our deeper truth in the midst of challenging circumstances. But then, this is part of what the spiritual path is about.

Creating material support for a spiritually integrated life involves integrating our temporal and spiritual life. Yet, there are times when we have to neglect our financial comfort in order to have the time to practice, or to learn to trust the moment-to-moment perfection of life. This is an area where Whitecloud and myself have put ourselves on the line countless times, sometimes having only a little food to eat and no where to sleep other than the ground. Yet in these circumstances we have received some of our most majestic empowerments.

Relationship

Relationship is an extremely important part of the spiritual path. It is a common occurrence that if one party of a relationship is growing and the other is not, that separation will most likely occur. It is not that each partner has to grow in exactly the same way or pace, rather that there is a certain dynamic that works.

There are three general approaches to our spiritual discovery. We totally depend on our own power such as in Zen, we totally depend on some other power such as a purely devotional path, or we work with a combination of our personal power and that of another being. Tantra is this third approach.

As we embrace the tantric path it is necessary to overcome the disempowerment of co-dependent relationships. It is a challenge to overcome co-dependency and yet honor our interactive oneness. As long as we feel trapped in karmic participation with our family and loved ones, we do not have the freedom to see from a wholistic perspective. Yogic practice gives us greater clarity to see. However, until we are familiar with the emptiness of form (a very primal experience), we are trapped in karmic participation no matter what we do. Relationship, and for that matter, everything, is a mirror. Lono, a Kahuna who lives in Crestone, Colorado, expounds a great wisdom in his saying, "that all we need as divine beings is a mirror." As we start to penetrate into a deeper reality, it is important that our intimate relationships are conducive to realization. This requires the recognition that our intimate partner(s) are our most intimate mirrors. Yet if we hang onto relation as our source, then we have mistaken the mirror for our source. The dynamics of intimate relationship are different for every person. For one person it may indicate a single committed relationship. For another, it may indicate staying free of committed relationships. There is no formula, only consciousness.

It is a great benefit to be with a partner who you can grow spiritually with in a positive, gentle, supportive relationship that simultaneously acknowledges the importance of overcoming karmic participation such as co-dependency, family and cultural conditioning, etc. This type of relationship will by the nature of two vital growing people be fiery at times and dynamic, so that energy is kept moving and stirring up what needs to be stirred up.

Right Diet

In addition to basic physical nutrition, food supports emotional habits, destroys or adds life force; in short it can hinder or support our clarity. Various foods can act as a conduit for subtle situations and entities, that until we gain mastery of, we need to be careful about eating those foods. I believe that a moderate, not too fussy diet is the best approach for most people.

I believe in a vegetarian diet, as this is a natural direction of refinement. Especially in today's easy abundance of food, there is no need to kill another being for food. Because you are not depending on the strength and emotional substance of an animal for your strength, you will have to find that strength more in yourself. This also gives you greater self-definition.

Exercise

I believe we all know the benefits of exercise and the good feeling it gives us, even if it is difficult for some of us to engage in much of it. Breathing, movement, dynamic yoga, walking, connecting to nature, and creating positive energetic guidelines to live by all supports greater clarity and thus spiritual progress.

Having a friend or place to go to (such as yoga classes) helps many in becoming more physically fit. Almost any inroad will open the doors to other inroads. For example, going on more frequent walks and hikes, or working out at the gym, or going to regular dynamic yoga classes, will increase our level of fitness to a point where it is easier to engage in other areas that we may have previously thought of as difficult.

This book has a number of dynamic yoga sets that will increase both a level of outer fitness, and because they are inherently directed in a manner of inner awareness, they will clear the body of agitations, so as to make it easier for us to meditate within our bodies as a support to greater spiritual awareness.

Becoming Happy

Becoming happy is becoming spiritually aware, becoming a whole human being that supports life, overcoming the bubble of separate existence and empowering the source of life.

In purifying ourselves we let go of our heaviness and what is not ours. Connect to what you really want and you naturally will become happier. It goes without saying that someone who listens to their soul will basically be happier than someone who is cut off from themselves.

A positive, life affirming attitude is essential for the tantric path, as happiness, pleasure and bliss are cultivated and used on this path. A negative, grumpy, depressed mode of life shuts down the basic disposition needed for the tantric path. A life-affirming disposition tends to embrace everything as part of the spiritual path, which is what tantra is about. A positive framework has the tenacity to go through all the ups and downs, and can make light of situations, and thereby see the underlying wisdom inherent in the constant reflection that life gives us.

Some of us only know happiness through feelings of power gained through exertion or command, but it does not last. This mimics happiness because there is a certain temporary centering in being successful. Happiness is something that may be triggered or enhanced by an outer experience, but lasting happiness itself is for no reason at all, other than the joy of life and love. In happiness our life force rests within our heart and radiates out. Intensified, this becomes bliss, and matured this becomes liberation.

Trying to intensify happiness through pumping lots of energy into the physical heart area can, if you are not careful, actually create difficulty in the body, such as chest problems. Happiness is a natural state that occurs through having a good disposition, purity, and letting go of contraction, not from grasping at it. As an example, it is better to cultivate happiness through an enjoyable walk in nature, working with our body in a friendly way such as yoga, helping a friend, having a good time, doing good work, feeling love for others, being kind and gentle to ourselves and others, calming the mind and letting it rest in the heart, eating the right foods, getting enough sleep, being positive, etc., rather than a concerted effort of "trying" to feel and collect happiness in our hearts.

Bliss, however can be and is intensified through yogic technique, because in these techniques we are beyond trying to create happiness per se, rather we create energy, blend it to suspend ourselves in a delicate and effortless balance and thereby penetrate into the natural bliss of our being. Bliss is the great consumer of the mind, emptying it of concerns and leaving it in its natural condition. While we must work to obtain the penetration that reveals bliss, we must not suffocate what it reveals to us in the fanaticism of our effort. This takes time, as at first we need that one-pointed concentration, and then we learn how to relax that concentration in an ever-expanding effortless and yet precise awareness.

Attitude and Commitment

Obviously without a commitment to developing inner awareness and bliss, nothing much will happen. However, there is an art in how to actualize our commitment into a support structure including supportive habits. Some suggestions in creating a workable structure for practice are given in later chapters of the book and much more can be given by a teacher over a period of time.

For those who are intense and total enough, they can create a blessed and somewhat fanatical beginning in which their lives totally revolve around yogic techniques. This is how I did it, and I highly recommend this path to those who are suited for it (yes I also worked for a living). However, this is only a first step, as what use is 6 or 16 hours of practice a day if that is the only way we can experience our divinity, eventually the situation changes and we are left high and dry if we have not discovered the innate divinity of our natural condition. And what about those who will practice for 30 minutes or an hour a day (I am sure there are many who are nodding their heads, and yes there is great benefit from 30 minutes a day.)

This is where commitment and a positive attitude comes in. After the romance (and during it as well), we have moments that are easier and moments that are not so easy. Moments when bliss flows as an effortless stream and moments when it is tough. Times when there is no time left for us. And for those of us who never got the initial romance, they will have to start with this aspect earlier with less background to draw upon. What is the secret?

The secret may sound like a religious sermon, but simply truth is truth. When we practice for the benefit of others and not just ourselves, this carries our practice forwards and guides it to adapt to the situation at hand. This is not just for a temporary benefit, a way to keep going, rather it is also grounded in our innate nature. Simply, we are all of each other and this is a doorway which if we ignore, we will miss the path to our full awakening, i.e., gaining definition within the body of oneness.

Practicing for the benefit of others has a passive side and an active side. Neither should overtake the other beyond the wisdom of the moment. For example we can within ourselves never want to hurt anyone, to pray that all beings are blessed, yet sometimes we need to see other sides of ourselves. These moments can be so strong that they overtake the pictures we want to paint in our mind, in order that we may understand these aspects and to really get a feel for owning our experiences and going deeper with them. They will happen anyway, but it is better if we can benefit by them. Sorrow, pain, disappointment, fear, anger are all great blessings on the path, if and only if we can take it into ourselves and for our own benefit blend into emptiness, understand the wisdom and for the benefit of others eventually elevate each experience. Then the spiritual path becomes alive and unstoppable. Practice becomes a way of staying connected, of deepening, and developing the continuum. When this continuum deepens, bliss results.

Be practical in your practice for the benefit of others. You are useless to others in a heavy confused state of being, and you help others in a bright happy state of mind even if you do your best to avoid them. Dedicate little moments, a smile, a friendly thought, an intention. These little moments, just like all the little moments of practice build, one upon the other and create an overall ambience. I have gotten through some of my most difficult times by deciding that the world had enough unhappiness in it, enough pain. When feeling the pain of others and then how my pain just adds to it all, my pain just simply had to give way. Give it a try next time you are in such a state.

Often, when reflecting on what I need to be for my full ascension in the bigger picture, it seems impossible. Sure I experience incredible states and what some would call siddha. I have that indescribable inner presence beyond form that is with me 24 hours a day, when I sleep, when I meditate, when I talk, and still it seems impossible to bring it into its full fruition through all the moments of the day. Then I reflect on all the help and resonance I get from masters who have achieved this, every day. I reflect on all the help I have given my incarnation from places beyond time and space. I feel the natural state and I remember the momentum and feel the reality, and I know it is unstoppable, greater than any outer force which could be imagined. This is why it is so important for those who want to go all the way that they develop a relationship with a teacher and with the masters. You thereby enter into a lineage of momentum, with vast reserves of talent, wisdom, love and help contained within it. Without this, it is indeed impossible, this is not something we can do by ourselves or only for ourselves, yet we are the ones who need to hold the primary responsibility, to do our practice when we do not feel like it, and to hold within the glimmers of truth that sustain us. This help is a thousand times more important than whatever level we think we have, or actually have achieved, even at the highest levels, we can go nowhere, in terms of the highest attainments, without it. This is not a law someone made up, just waiting for the first being to overcome it. It simply results from the reality of the body of the one, interdependence, ati, or the sameness of form and emptiness as the Buddhist say.

As part of your commitment, it is highly recommended that you create periods of intensive practice in your life, i.e., retreats. It is during these times that you will most likely really get the taste, really experience yourself as a divine being. Of course the first few retreats might be time off, might be purification and healing, or learning how to meditate better. But keep in mind that as we become more skillful in applying ourselves that a retreat is not just time off, rather it has only one purpose which is to overcome our conditioned view of reality. It takes the intense focus of a retreat practice to go through the initial uncomfortableness of loosing our regular concrete sense of identity so that we may discover ourselves in innate effortless radiance and wisdom. As a retreat builds, or after a few of them, a day of this preciousness might seem like a year of regular practice. First get yourself to a place where you can apply yourself in such a way, pray for it, get some help from a teacher, and then just do it.

In regards to our attitude, well a good attitude will work wonders and a rotten attitude spoils everything. It is fine and dandy to say, I will always have a great attitude towards life, but this requires a commitment to being clear. Creating and maintaining clarity is a fruit of yogic practice, so there are tools we can use to achieve this. At some point, however always trying to maintain a good attitude gives way to just being natural, because we are interdependent beings, and if we try too hard not to reflect those around us and our own condition, this can also become a trap. So we do our best, continue doing our best, but we let go of any heavy attitude about it. Bliss has a wonderful way of removing the ambition of attitude.

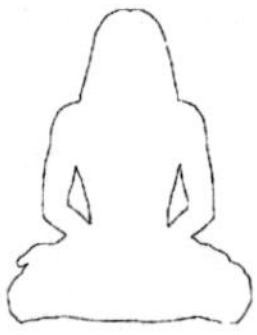

3

Introduction To Yogic Preliminary Practices

A Foundation for Success

Preliminary practices create a strong foundation for spiritual success. **Any cultivation that re-orientates us from a mundane outlook into our spiritual brilliance and beauty can be thought of as a preliminary practice.** Thus it is important not to confuse the word "preliminary" with something that we quickly outgrow, or do not need to pursue because we are so great. Think of preliminary, as that which precedes the fullness of our accession. Preliminary practices are skillful means, and there are many of them. There are practices to suit every kind of temperament, cultivations to suit those who do not like the idea of a fixed regime, and places to start for those who do not know where to start. This book does not attempt to give methods for every temperament, rather it is written for those who like the effectiveness, bliss, and rich flavor of the disciplined yogic path.

A Practice as it evolves, is more than some mechanical repetition of a mantra, breath, movement, or focus. It is the enjoyment of finding and then remaining in our blissful center. Repetition, when made alive, brings us through our constant need of need, of grasping for outer stimulation, and enters us into our eternal place of fulfillment. We break out of the prison of our self-pettiness and enter the vastness of whom we really are. It is practice in the sense that we need practice to build focus, we need practice at applying our focus, and we need experience to know how to do it.

Repetition builds the potency of what starts as mundane speech, mundane breath, mundane movement, mundane thinking, and refines this into ecstatic beingness radiating through word, thought, and movement.

Yoga begins by emphasizing and building a positive and thus radiant outlook. A positive outlook teaches us that life is what we choose to make out of it. We turn towards the great perfection. This attitude is the initial understanding of emptiness, which is at the very core of more advanced practices. A positive state of consciousness is an aspect of radiance, and radiance in its refinement is spirit. The nature of spirit itself is radiant emptiness. Emptiness as a descriptive word is a crude attempt at describing this richness without boundaries, which may also be termed a primal oneness. Yet with all its misunderstood connotations, emptiness is still one of the best starting points to be cognitive of our unlimited nature. A positive person has a good-natured compassionate disposition. A positive disposition springs forth from valuing radiance, which again is also at the core of spiritual practice. Valuing the clarity of radiance is what creates the necessity of doing elevating practices. As we progress, these aspects enliven us to the entire essence of creation: emptiness and form.

Yogic techniques increase our voltage and clarity, which supports a positive nature. We clear away toxins, neurosis and confusion. While this requires discipline, as it catches, and we apply ourselves, we are carried in a momentum. In the process we discover ourselves, and this renewal is precious. As we value clarity, the yogic techniques become a way of entering, maintaining, and getting back this clarity. It is not about eastern or western, mysticism or scientifism; rather it is practical and sacred application of ourselves. As we learn how to unite our body, breath and mind as a single sacred activity, then the bounds of what is thought of as yoga loosens, and we are able to apply the strength and beauty of our body, mind and breath in all sorts of activities.

Yoga is scholarly defined as something like "union," or to join our higher and lower self. In twenty years of practicing and teaching various yogas, I never thought of yoga in that way. This type of definition, while incredibly profound in its highest meaning, in practicality can easily become too dictionary like and steeped in separation. For me Yoga, even if it is not the dictionary meaning of the word, is the skillful ways of applying ourselves into greater clarity and presence. Rather than a noun, yoga is a verb. In that clarity, union is already there and we just expand our vista of it. Thus yoga is an activity in which we find ourselves.

If Yoga is to be true in this way, then it has to promote integration with movement and life. By varying our emphasis between depth and movement we create a dynamic of consciousness that does not grasp at itself. In the process we see and address our issues. While this requires grit, the renewal that results makes it invaluable. To empower grit, we inspire ourselves with possibilities: friends who are also doing these practices, a teacher who lives for this, illuminating stories of various practitioners and our own dreams. **Mostly, we inspire ourselves through the necessity of practice.** Perhaps we are a little gullible or fanatical at first, miss a key point for a while, exaggerate a bit here, or create a prop over there; but we know that our pure inner essence, such as in the quiet moments, will direct us forward.

It is this confidence and lack of doubt which yoga instills that warms us to greater possibility. After all, the silky-like delicate embrace, the tingling sensations, the potency, the quieting of our mind and the indescribable inner-space that opens up is experiential. It is similar to a bunch of people debating whether out-of-body experiences are a figment of the imagination, and then you have one; end of debate. You no longer have time for such intellectuality, for there is a grand world awaiting us within and reflecting all around us. Life becomes precious.

The techniques presented here are invaluable and extremely precious in creating a foundation for tantric practices. The difference between yogic and tantric practice is as much the internal development of the practitioner as the technique itself. For a person who has matured into tantric practice, the yogic techniques are a secondary support means of the primary tantric practices. Tantric practices are much more direct in that the technique is in essence connectivity with our true nature. In the highest level of practice, all techniques are a secondary support to the actuality of being consciously conscious twenty-four hours a day.

Thus techniques will not of themselves bring you ascension, but they greatly help us to get there. Treat them as good friends and keep consistent company with their benefits, like a drowning man or woman would of a rope thrown in the water for him or her to grasp hold of.

Structured techniques require us to apply ourselves in ways that build the understanding, grounding and strength necessary to correctly meditate. Free-flow meditation is beyond the necessity of an artificially created support structure and thus very creative in nature. Passive meditation only yields fruit when two simultaneous and indivisible qualities are present: radiance and emptiness. We are simply aware of emptiness and form in a non-dualistic radiant manner. Activity and form is the radiant aspect (effortless consciousness) of emptiness. Active techniques develop self-definition, which is another way of saying that we have the ability to stay awake in our deepening penetration. This wakefulness is supported by unconditional radiance. The form our meditation takes in any given moment should be self-obvious. If we put too much emphasis on emptiness meditation before we have enough self-definition (radiance), before we are present enough, then we simply fall asleep. Nothing is gained of much value.

The word "passive" in passive mediation may be a little misleading to someone wanting an undisciplined easy way out. Passive meditation is only practical when you are grounded within the aliveness of the inner core of your body. The word passive refers to the impossibility of obtaining Buddhahood through techniques, rather, it is our primal-awareness itself, and the continuity of remaining in this through every form and nuance that is being referred to. The word passive also refers to the true creative sense of space, beyond a grasping of self, in which everything exists.

A Kriya is an active type of technique, rather than a passive approach. If passive meditation brings forth the image of looking at a wall and becoming blank, then you are advised to practice kriya instead. Also, if you think that passive meditation is a way to become enlightened through using your un-enlightened mind, then you definitely should start with kriya. Remember that we get there by being there.

Kriyas often involve a combination of connected visualization, breathing and posture or movement to create a presence that is automatically meditative and nonverbal. When the presence does not easily come forth, then kriya creates a pressure, which by remaining within, eventually leads to effortless presence. Kriyas create energy to support awakening consciousness and a pathway to draw our rebellious and outward seeking mind into the quietude and awareness of our inner sanctum. Thus kriyas often contain creative variations, according to the type of energy created and how much activity is needed to create that energy. For example, a beginning practitioner may fall asleep or become distracted trying to practice a very subtle kriya that does not use the breath or a mind-capturing movement.

Kriyas give way over years of practice to a natural meditation within the core of our being, but even then it is wise to keep one or two of them active for the purpose of greater integration, aliveness of being, and to share with others.

Dynamic Yoga sets are combinations of postures and movements that are vitalizing, activating, purifying and centering in nature. They are a type of Kriya that is movement meditation with lots of spirit. Another name for Dynamic Yoga is Kundalini Yoga. Kundalini is the emotional-energy-substance moving through our body that blends subtle awareness with our body and enlivens the whole yogic experience.

Dynamic Yoga is an excellent way to purify, heal, and prepare us for deeper meditation. This type of movement, while perhaps a bit difficult at first because of sore muscles, is like dance. Dance is nonverbal, connected, sensual, ecstatic (or at least fun), and beautiful. It is a meditation in itself that evaporates sluggishness of mind and body.

In yogic practices we are not so concerned about the content of our feelings. We do not try to constantly figure out why we feel up or down, sad or happy; rather we wash and elevate ourselves into simple radiant nonverbal presence. Being able to continually come back into this state is a key for consistent spiritual development. Becoming familiar with our radiant presence will help us to take responsibility for what we create in our life. This will enhance the ability to master our thoughts and subtle projection through discrimination and positivity.

Thus a keynote of this stage of practice is moving energy (emotions, blockages, toxins, grasping, etc.,) and making enough voltage to feel radiant and empowered to move in response to our higher calling.

As we advance in our Kriya practice we learn how to condense and contain large amounts of prana within both our physical and subtle bodies, and in the process totally open and vitalize all the channels of the body. Nectar is created and held within the protective womb of the body's inner core that supports our blissfully radiant awareness in everyday life, thus the term, nectar body. This creates the necessary potency for the tantric expansion and blending of the advanced practices. Without this vitality, it is like trying to run on slippery ice, there simply is not enough traction long enough to get a grip and it seems hopeless to reach our destination.

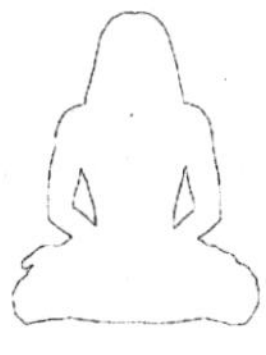

4

Role of a Teacher

For most of the practices presented in this book a teacher (or teachers) is highly recommended and very helpful, but not absolutely necessary for everyone. It depends on your background, natural understanding, and how far you want to go.

In regards to the actual techniques, some people pick them up quickly while others need more help in regards to the subtlety. A teacher helps with this by giving a feeling of the practice, and a good teacher can transmit (as appropriate) to receptive and ready students a temporary experience of how energy flows in the body while doing a practice.

For many practitioners, after about six months (more or less), everything is going well and then they hit a wall. That is, emotions come up, it is difficult and distractions present themselves. This is a point where a teacher can really help. This is in reference to someone who is really qualified to work with people in this way, in contrast to a technician, who may be good at showing the yogic techniques, but not so intuitive and skilled in the deeper currents. The teacher tells you to keep going through it even though you may not feel like it. A teacher can give you some feedback as to what is occurring.

For myself, after about eight months of intense practice, I felt like my heart was being pulled out of me. Sometimes I would silently cry for half an hour before starting my late evening kriya, and then when I started, I would become extremely blissful. In short I felt like I was being wrung through a washing machine. My teacher at that time simply put me on a three-week juice fast, and everything came right.

During this time, I learned how to create bliss, but my attachment to it made the cycles of cleansing much more difficult. My energy was penetrating into the inner channels, but was not yet stabilized, nor was there enough wisdom to understand the intricacies. Sometimes, I would try to trace an emotion to some past occurrence or thought, and so on, to try to find its source (which seemed endless, one thing leads to the next). Much of the time, my mind would devotionally, yet sometimes mechanically, silently chant a mantra (Sat Naam) for many hours at a time. Finally I figured out what that mantra meant. If I was cold and I thought to be warm, that is Sat Naam. Even if that thought did not immediately create warmth, non-the-less it is just a matter of time and cultivation. Acknowledging I was warm, even when I was not, and relaxing my mind not to think otherwise, is Sat Naam. It does not matter about the endless content; it is the qualifying ability of the radiant-mind that is Sat Naam[1]. That realization enabled a force within me to bring an end to the washing machine effect.

A teacher can help keep you on track, so that you make these kinds of discoveries for yourself. One of the primary roles of a teacher is to return students to themselves, so they understand for themselves the effect of what they create and where they are going.

A teacher can protect you to a certain degree through this time, provided you listen. This activity occurs both in subtle activity and through outward advice, such as doing a certain practice, being careful at a certain time, or to do a certain activity in order to mitigate something else. For example, one of our students about a decade ago was very eager and excited at what was occurring for him. I said to him, that in so many months time, he was going to challenge us, and the choice he would make at that time was very crucial. Well, nothing was pointing that way in the moment, so I think he forgot about it.

So many months later to the very day, an event occurred which he thought was unfair and he did challenge us. He was very sure of himself and that would have been the last we heard of him, except I called him that night and reminded him of what I said so many months previously. It was like the straw that broke the camels back, and he broke down and had a huge healing. Because a teacher has had a lot of personal experience, these things are seeable and somewhat predictable. So a teacher can help return a student to himself or herself in the delicate and tricky arena of the psyche.

A teacher can transmit or help you to remember certain depths. Often, the receptivity and possibility of these experiences are created through the kriyas and yoga. Thus while a practitioner does not necessarily need a teacher to benefit from these practices, a teacher can deepen those practices greatly. Many of the experiences I had in my early years of kriya, were remarkable, enlightened states of mind. It would take me many more years to recognize them for what they were and to stabilize those experiences, but nevertheless they created a seed.

I believe that many sincere practitioners have these types of experiences early on. There is a certain innocence that allows it. As

1 Its literal Translation is Truth (Sat) is my name (Naam), i.e., my true identity. For me, this truth is radiance from deep within, thus I would think of Sat Naam as I Am Radiant. I later understood it more fully as the indivisible reality of emptiness (Sat) and form or identity (Naam). This mantra also balances the elements of the body allowing an effortless blending of identity with the oneness or emptiness that is the basis of all reality.

we become more sophisticated in our knowledge, we tend to forget the grace that comes with pure innocence. This is a stage that must be gone through.

Yoga and Kriyas require a grounding to bear fruit, and this takes awhile. For a serious practitioner who wants to go all the way, it is often beneficial if it takes a while. Otherwise the practitioner grounds the practice through a type of egotistical previously attained grounding.

While this is not a path for the timid, through intensity we somewhat blow ourselves apart. There is no ground to stand on. For myself, a few times this became quite literal as I watched the ground underneath me become light; there was no up or down, in or out. Often when I came out of napping, I could not remember my name or where I was, other than I had dissolved very, very deep. I was forced to find my identity again from that very deep place and eventually bring it into a continuum. At that time I had no idea of the specifics, but now I recognize this as part of the traditional preparation for the tantras.

There is a time, which most kriya practitioners go through, when the sexual force that is transmuted starts to build and swell in the back of the head. When this is combined with kriya, you can become a bit spacey for a few months[1]. You are in a very nonverbal state that sees things differently than most people. A teacher can recognize these places, and encourage you through them, rather than to fall back on worldly ideas. Later the integration will come, but sometimes it is good to blast things apart a little bit. Later this proves invaluable in being ready to partake of the higher paths, such as the tantras. Otherwise, it is unlikely you will enter these paths correctly because there remains too much limited identity within relationship, security, personality, etc.

Seemingly unfair things can and do happen to us on the spiritual path and it is all perfect. This is part of your surrender and trust. As I said in the beginning, it is up to you how far you want to go and

1 I can hear some people saying there are easy fixes for these states in terms of circulating energy, but that presumes a grounding and a much more gradual path. Grounding is definitely necessary for every stage of the path, but when it is done from the place of "no ground," this has tremendous benefits. This does not mean a lack of bodily connectivity; in fact it increases it in the long term. Also there has to be a certain amount of energy circulation for these states to even occur. It is not simply a stagnation of energy in the back of the head, or some other area of the body, but a clearing of major and minor channels into a deeper place.

how fast. It is enough for most just to practice the kriyas and yoga to feel good and be more efficient and happy in what they do. This is a fine motivation. But in terms of the big picture, it is also a much more gradual approach. Intensity is not something that you force, but it births from inside of you at the right times. Life's opportunities are precious.

Another, potentially tricky area is sexual energy. Most practices (unless it has been neutered) will increase your sexual energy. This is very important. Along with this increase, we learn how to use this energy as basic life force to enliven and support our spiritual growth. This energy can become so universal in how it is used, that some people simply call it life force and leave out the sexual qualification.

Problems arise when we do not know how to contain or properly use this energy. All sorts of projections can occur and relationships can become confused. It is very important for us to be intimate within ourselves, yet we do not always feel comfortable being honest with ourselves. In one way we are dissolving limitations and in another way we need to honor boundaries and fortify them.

Burning out grosser sexual currents created by misunderstanding and toxins is a time of purification and transmutation. It is not a time to engage sexually, because you will only reinforce old habits. While some can work this out for themselves, a teacher helps bring clarity at this time.

Having a teacher is not about giving your power away; rather it is a sacred relationship where you become empowered. Surrender is important, provided the main surrender is the chitchat mind and its righteousness. This is what kriya does anyway; thus for someone who is really practicing, it is not an issue. A teacher is not someone who will do everything for you, but will help the "feeling," also called "transmission," of achievement. There are a lot of fine corrections along the way. A teacher can draw attention to these. A skilled teacher will however, mostly, clothe those corrections in a way where you have to apply yourself and thus jointly discover their value for yourself. Sometimes this is very blunt and straightforward, such as "get off of it." Then you have to figure how to get of off it, yet when you surrender, you already know. In the end, there is no one to complain to.

Later, in the tantras, the role of a teacher becomes much more central. These first stages are a training ground where you learn what this relationship is and is not.

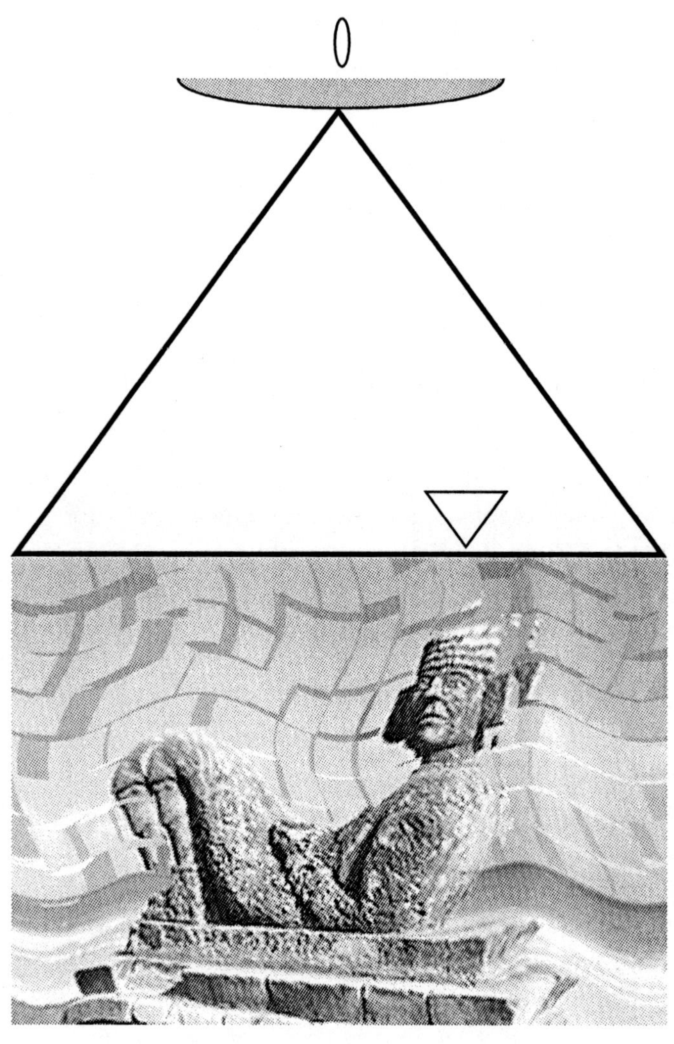

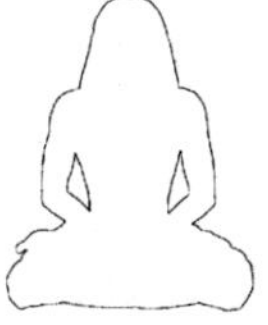

5

Guidelines for Practice

Establishing a Practice

Setting the Energy and Dedicating our Practice

Pacing Ourselves

Women and their Menstruation

Moving Through Resistance into Benefit

Composure

Some ABC's of the Yogic Path

A Progression of Techniques

Establishing a Practice

The degree of benefit obtained from these practices depends on what you want, your willingness to move in that direction, and the developed skill of that application.

These practices nurture something within us that feels great, bringing forth clarity, beauty, vitality, dynamic peace, and a spacious nonverbal awareness from within. Sometimes it is first caught from being around other people who hold that energy, and then you take it from there, developing it for yourself. Mostly it is a day-to-day deepening through the empowerment of consistency. This benefit compounds upon itself, because we are now better able to grow from life's outer reflections, activities, and challenges.

For a lasting benefit you must apply yourself daily. Commit to what you can honestly do every day without overstressing yourself. You may want to do additional practices for fun, but keep the committed practice every day. For example, you may decide to commit to the SaTaNaMa kriya everyday for six weeks, yet do other practices most of the time.

Men and women tend to approach spiritual discipline in different ways. It is more important for a man to keep a certain practice every day for the committed time no matter what. Women tend to need "some" flexibility. This is a reflection of internal chemistry and differences between the feminine and masculine.

When our practice becomes the *Yoga of Necessity,* only then does it really catch. Previous to this, yoga and kriyas are just something else to do and like any fad, after awhile we loose interest in it. It is not until we value our clarity so much so, that to loose it is a spiritual death. This intensity and passion of yoga enables us to maintain and regain clarity amidst the dynamic of life. As we gain confidence in our clarity: grasping ceases, we open up (in the free-flow of love), non-conceptuality arises and we may mature into the tantric path[1].

To value clarity requires wisdom. For example, if we feel that our efforts in worldly-activity is enough in itself to enter real clarity, then we do not yet understand the yoga of necessity; "If I simply had more money, then I could meditate," or "its not yet time (because of other things I must do in the world)." For a yogi, these techniques are their

1 The tantric path encompasses and elevates all of our innate qualities, such as desire and aggression, to unveil the freedom of non-dualistic consciousness that is effortless even amidst effort.

lifeline. We are swimming in a huge sea, and that rope is all there is between unconscious ignorance and being consciously conscious. At the same time, if we do not learn to swim in unconditional luminosity (through the aid of the practices), we will eventually drown anyway. **Thus the yoga of necessity is the absolute necessity to deal with the world in radiant perspective and not drown in its apparent density.** It is the desire to be happy because there is already too much unhappiness in the world. It is the desire to be clear because there is already too much confusion in the world. This desire is what makes the yoga — necessary. In that instant of pure motivation, clarity shines through, and we regain our inner-radiance at all costs. When we are in danger, it is no time to think about other things; we must remain present and alert. When you loose clarity, no one cares about the reason why; you must regain it. This is the realness, sink or swim, of the spiritual path

As you advance in your practice, it is the essence which is important, and thus your practice may stick to a certain form or not, depending on what you or your teacher knows best at that time.

Early in the morning, before the sun rises, is always a great time to meditate. This is very practical in regards to daytime jobs. Always meditate before going to sleep, even if just for a few minutes; consistency is the key.

Sooner or later in the daily practice of a particular kriya a point is reached where no further growth appears to be coming forth from the practice; it kind of goes flat. It is your trust in the technique or your teacher to keep practicing anyway. This usually occurs within three weeks to two months. This is a crucial time.

The assistance of an experienced teacher is invaluable, as the teacher can help you to understand if you should move on to another technique, or stay with it. Much of this is determined by if the technique is a preliminary preparation, or if it has the personal potential to bring you right into your depth. A teacher can remind you of motivation, which when sparked, gives that little extra to elevate a technique from being mechanical to an exquisite experience. A teacher can also recognize when a students resistance, known or unknown, toxic, emotional, from whatever reason, personal or environmental, is making practice difficult and apparently unfruitful.

This period is an opportunity to bring forth our creative essence, which is what practice is about. In the beginning of a practice, we are motivated by the possibility it presents and in the challenge of its mastery. There is a certain aliveness of creative essence that fuels us. As time continues, some of that initial enthusiasm may become dampened and the practice becomes a routine. As practitioners, we must now penetrate past the routine into our core radiance and awareness, which when connected with, makes any practice or activity enjoyable and profound. The practice must seduce us into an enlightened sphere of awareness.

Setting the Energy and Dedicating your Practice

It is helpful to have a place in your house or room where you practice. Make an alter and keep the area clean. If it is in your living room, place a cloth over the TV.

Doing a particular practice at the same time everyday creates a habit that makes the practice easier to continue on days when you do not feel like it. It is a way of saying this is a priority in my life.

Before you begin, sit or stand for a few minutes, center yourself, set your intention and dedicate the practice for something good. Sometimes, when the mood strikes, I put on appropriate, lively music and dance. I dance energy, love, excitement, prayer in all directions, feeling it spread and uplift people. Then I settle into a yoga set. By dedicating the good energy and realizations resulting from your practice for the benefit of others, the positive energy is anchored into a larger field that uplifts other people and creates a grace that will benefit you during future practice. Perhaps feel or visualize a blessing light spreading in all directions, connecting to anyone who needs or attunes with the good energy you are creating.

This type of dedication often results in the first conscious moments of connecting into the sambhogakaya (soul) and dharmakaya (spirit) realms for a practitioner. Anchoring your practice through a sincere heart-felt radiant blessing prayer for all beings carries the benefits of practice forward from one session to the next so that it builds. Without this anchoring, the benefits received can easily dissipate during the day and we are continually starting from scratch. In more advanced practices it often results in ten to a hundred times the difference of what is achieved over the years.

When you finish a session, never just jump up. Rather seal the energy first through a dedication or prayer. A wonderful way is to place the hands together in prayer pose at the heart and chant long Sat Naam's for three or more times. Inhale deep and chant in a long drawn out way "Saaaat," then (in the same breath) "Naaam" in a lower tone and drawn out but not as long as the "Sat." "Sat" rhymes with "but." Naam is pronounced as in Viet-naam. Chant it in a way that resonates inside your torso and simultaneously feel ever-opening circles of blessing presence moving into the world. This will give you a relationship with the mantra while subtly expressing your sacred energy.

For those who have begun the Eternal Yoga practices, after you do your dedication at the end of a session, go above the head and make the intention that the positive energy from this session will act throughout your day and that any realizations and cultivations will remain intact until your next session[1]. This is not so much a prayer, but a visualization that holds an intention beyond outer disturbance and the effects of time and space. This only takes a few minutes, but again, can save you years of floundering and builds a sacred momentum that keeps your practice alive. For a busy man or woman in today's world it is essential, as we do not always have the immediate time to meditatively build upon a subtle insight or revelation in our meditation.

Pacing Ourselves in Practice

In regards to physical exercises, such as in the dynamic yoga sets, start gradually in the beginning so as to allow your muscles and physiology to adjust. Keep in mind that there are times when you need to blast through, or to shift, an emotion or mindset, and a good sweaty workout can do just that. Fitness is not just muscular, but also largely measured by how well you can remain present in what you are doing (with enjoyment). If your mind is constantly wandering, work to keep it contained using breath, intention, exercise and grounding.

1 By very consciously going above the head and making an imagined continuum of that awareness from the present sitting to the next sitting, it is kept alive in its original essence. When you next sit, as you deepen in awareness, it will reappear for further exploration and integration.

In the dynamic yoga sets each exercise is typically done for 1 to 3 minutes. Some people, as they warm up to it over the weeks or months, extend these times, while another person may only be able to do an exercise for a much shorter time. What works for you is the correct time. Generally, the exercises are done in synch with the breath, so obviously we move at a pace in which our breath can keep up. There are some exceptions to this (these are stated).

Deep breathing is used in almost all the exercises. As you can breathe deeply and easily, then this somewhat exaggerated breath brings in more energy than the body needs. Through staying present, the extra prana is distilled from the breath and condensed into the inner spaces of the body. This takes time to understand and to clear your energy channels so this can occur. If you get dizzy, the above is not happening. Slow down or stop and pace yourself accordingly. Make sure that you are always breathing down into your navel or lower abdomen.

After building soft energy through meditation, sometimes squeeze various muscles to force the energy deeper into the body and to help contain it. This is a tremendous energy tonic. It clears the channels and grounds us in our bodies. This can be used a the end of a sitting pranayama, a standing martial arts stance, or whenever it seems beneficial

In Dynamic Yoga, flexibility is secondary and not strived for beyond a reasonable amount. More important is obtaining a connectivity of body, mind, and breath. This connectivity is what allows physical yoga exercises to become movements of our soul.

In regards to how long to practice a sitting kriya or meditation; general guidelines are given with each practice. For a pranayama, 10 minutes is a good time to start with, which is gradually built upon. Chants and silent practices are usually done for 30 minutes to start with. If this is too much, start with 15 minutes and gradually build your time.

Dizziness or becoming spacey is a sign that our energy is not yet able to move through the appropriate channels. Heart palpitations or heaviness result from too much energy getting caught up in the chest, most often from incorrect breathing or practice. All these are signs to stop for the moment, stretch a bit or walk around, and in general to go more slowly. As we gradually progress, our energy channels become clear and our capacity thus increases. No benefit is obtained from stressing ourselves out in a practice. These blockages can be from toxins, emotional charge, physical difficulties, and simply lack of use.

If you have a physical disability whereby you cannot apply this type of exercise, do not feel disheartened, for there are many types of practice still available to you, such as visualization. Remember soft energy is unlimited and can be worked with in unlimited quantities. Our refinement into soft, alive, and unlimited energy is a much greater strength than most people realize.

In silent sitting meditation without a particular form, sit through initial distractions and then as long as desired. If you are too heady, bring your focus down into the lower body with the aid of your breath. If you are drowsy, either do some breathing exercises or meditate at the third eye point. Generally in this kind of meditation, we move through a number of plateaus. Thus we may stretch a bit or take a brief walk in-between these plateaus, without letting our mind become too external. In this way we maintain freshness and naturalness without abandoning our inner movement.

If you are very tired, do not push yourself. Rather surrender into that tiredness and simply observe it. See where you are. You may surprise yourself how much you internally wake up. Otherwise either take a shower and start again, or sit for a few minutes and go to sleep. Never, ever push yourself in a direction that increases internal pain, headiness or heaviness . Neither should you be too timid in your practice. Again a teacher is of help. This is fanaticism and is of no benefit. Get advice from a teacher for more specifics into a reoccurring theme of this nature.

For beginners, dynamic movement often brings a deeper experience of integration and meditation than still practice. At this stage of practice, one of the maxims is moving energy. Thus if nothing is happening in still meditation, shift into something that moves energy, such as breath of fire. Then sit. We need that voltage.

For experienced practitioners, it is important to extend kriyas and silent meditations for longer times. When it becomes effortless to practice for increasingly longer times, this corresponds to certain energy breakthroughs in the physical and subtle body. A substance has been cultivated in the body that supports subtle awareness. When you are able to remember where you have been and what has occurred in your deeper sittings to the level of the dream body, corresponding to the throat chakra, this makes it easy to sit through the forty minute to one-hour barrier. Sitting effortlessly and focused for two hours or longer indicates that your energy is able to move into the deeper channels of the subtle-body and simultaneously you are more connected to you inner earth aspect. Properly meditating for three hours or longer is a definite opening within one or more chakras along with a whole-body circulation.

Longer meditations are difficult or impossible without being comfortably grounded within the inner essence of our body. Longer meditation results from an effortlessness that is supported by a fine prana. This prana originates most easily though the inner core of our body. If we are not grounded within our core, then we are not remaining in this prana. Even when we become transcendent of the body, this is achieved by going deeper into the inner channels, or within a prepared energy structure, not by spacing out. This inner grounding is very expansive. Even, when an experienced yogi has died, the body can remain upright and fresh for a few days or weeks, because they are still alive in the inner channels of the body. Then the outer body falls limp as they take that inner body elsewhere. Thus practice being present in your body as you do the kriyas. This will give a ten-fold increase in their power.

While a very advanced practitioner can go right into this core of fine prana, irrespective of their physical health, for most of us, the support for longer meditation comes from a mixture of this extremely fine prana and the subtle energy from our organs, tissues and environment. Thus, by gradually awakening each of our organs through breathing, positive emotion, and exercise, we gain support for longer wakeful practice.

Being present in our practice allows us to sit longer. It is not difficult to watch a two-hour TV program, because it captures our attention. Time is irrelevant. Similarly, when we are really present in our practice it is effortless. The most important moments of a chanting kriya are the first few minutes. If in this time, we really make an effort to be present (no excuses allowed) with what we are doing, in our bodies, and with an iron-presence not to allow our thoughts to drift, then that sets the direction. As our energy is going deeper through the chant, our awareness is right there with it. There is a unification of body, mind and energy. It is timeless and effortless, and this opens a corresponding inner space within the body. This creates a nonverbal strength of mind that supports our practice. However, if we are not with it, then as our energy is internalized, our mind is somewhere else. This creates a split, which is felt as distraction, boredom, or tiredness.

An experienced teacher or a fellow practitioner with considerable common-sense experience can show you how to properly pace yourself, and when it is appropriate to push yourself (such as moving through resistance).

A Woman on her Menstrual Cycle

A woman on her moon cycle, particularly in the heavier days, should only do light stretching. Do not apply muscular contractions (bhands), breath of fire, and any exercise where you hold or extend your breath. It is a time to go into the earth and a time to quietly see from within. A forcing of energy upwards will interfere with the normal downward flow at this time, and can create difficulties. There are exceptions to the above, as a yogic training to stop the moon cycle, but this is not advised for most people.

Besides a time of cleansing the blood, for some woman it is also a time of increased vision into what they need to see. Thus, far from being a disability in the continuum of practice, the monthly cycle can be a time of seeing through obstructions, gaining important insights and honoring connectivity, thus accelerating your practice. It is a time of the perfection of the body in its cycles, If you fight that perfection, by trying to ignore your moon cycle, you will be trying to fit your practice into a male orientated schedule which is not created for the feminine body. If you go with it, by being flexible in the nature of your practice and activities, you can advance as fast or faster than a man, while making it easier on yourself in the process.

Moving Through Resistance into Benefit

Spiritual practice will directly confront resistance. For a motivated person, the resistance to practice is not the real issue, although at times it may appear to be so. Rather, the resistance is to deep changes the practice creates or to the penetration it brings into seeing what does not want to be seen. This is a very common, predictable, and frequently occurring issue with most people who do spiritual practices, and even many who are advanced. The easier and more graceful way is to cut through the resistance with your practices combined with the willingness to see and grow. Otherwise, it becomes the school of hard knocks.

If there is a kriya or technique you find particularly beneficial or attractive, practice it for at least six weeks. This amount of time allows for the technique to move through the phases of your psyche. Thus there may be times where it is easy, times where it is not, times it gives a lot of energy, and times when their appears to be no benefit. In this way you "rewire" parts of yourself, move through any cloudy energy inside yourself, extend your subtle penetration, and integrate the practice to a deeper level.

Establishing connectivity (rewiring) and bringing up blockages and issues to be worked through can be much more intense than you may at first think. People often do not belief me when I say this, for they underestimate the power of what they are practicing. The better we practice, the more stuff gets dug up. This is why it is better to only commit to one or two practices and do the rest for fun. Otherwise, we may overburden ourselves and in response, not do anything. Of course this will bring an immediate benefit of relief, but it makes it more difficult in the long run to again bring up the issue and work through it. Remember, the only way out is through. Today is all you can truly count on.

Composure

The composure in which we move from one exercise to the next or how we majestically sit in meditation is of the utmost importance. For example, when you finish a difficult arm exercise, do not collapse, instead gracefully place your arms down, somewhat like a ballerina. Carry this presence from one exercise to the next. Collapsing at the end of an exercise reinforces a weak self-image and prevents the mastery of an exercise. If you need to stop or lie down, then do so gracefully.

Think of a yogi who sits through ups and downs, cold and heat with the presence of a king and the grace of radiance. Made of iron, flexible as a soft rose petal, with nothing to prove, he or she moves in response to the need, giving what arises from the nectar of their being.

The way in which we carry ourselves either strengthens or weakens our etheric image. This is not about stiffness and fanaticism, but a genuine cultivating of energy awareness. When we maintain and finish an exercise or kriya properly, our energy aligns into the channels of the body, and we remain in the after effect of the practice. We value what we are doing. This approach makes our practices many times more potent. It builds the type of energy where we can just about jump out of our skin, except the inner space is vaster, so instead of jumping out of our skin, we become multidimensional.

By being present and aware, we learn how to anchor within our bones and energy-flows, and from there into eternal radiance. Some people practice yoga for years and yet never experience a thoughtless mind and bliss. If you allow your mind to continually race elsewhere, your breath uncontrolled, your body to twitch and wriggle, your energy wanting to do something else; what do you expect? If you can practice with mindfulness, you will become more grounded, connected and present. In this you will be light, happy and free. The very motion of yoga becomes an enlightened activity. This is surrender.

Regality is head, heart, and navel combined as a whole to provide a venue for the soul to feel itself. This whole body feeling is automatically free of grasping. Regality is the opposite of the wandering mind and collapsing in the face of difficulty. It is something that is cultivated through sincerity and maturity, and expounded through the popular saying from Yogi Bhajan "Keep Up and you will be Kept Up." Applying a light Mhula-Bhand (see next chapter) from time to time while directing energy into wakefulness helps this feeling.

Regality is radiant clarity, which is another way of stating the indivisible awareness of emptiness and form. This consciousness, whether appearing withdrawn, outrageous, strong, or meek, always contains a kind of radiance that can only result from depth. We possess an enthusiasm that is married to a quietness of mind and thus there is no need to argue. Regality results from having some type of substance inside of us and awakening our radiance within that substance. It releases the sense of struggle through a command of lightness and upward flow of energy. This helps to seal the effect of the kriya or exercise by absorbing the soft pranas created into the tissues of the body, and to reinforce a feeling of clarity and strength. Neutrality is cultivated within the emotions, giving rise to higher emotion and the ability to be in the pure energy of emotion.

When our ego or invested identity is shattered; joy to the world, for we realize our eternalness and keep going from something inside that is always going. We are not so concerned with why we are neurotic, happy or sad; we simply wash, purify, and elevate everything constantly. We do not hide, rather we elevate. This is a direct confrontation to the ego, which wants to justify itself and play through our dramas. It is a great training for the tantras, and its emphasis on emptiness. It is said in Buddhist texts "that when emptiness appears, a hundred and twelve problems disappear." One second they define us, the next second they are … empty. For many, when they first feel the emptiness, as they arise from their meditation and enter the world they feel emotionally and physiologically empty and to the ever busy mind which must feel its mark on the world this is a greater problem than all their other problems. The solution is to keep going into it, so that you may find the true indivisible nature of emptiness and all of creation, i.e., richness.

There is a time when we must face and perfect all our neurosis into the ever-expanding perfection. This is the wisdom of the Mother. For this to be integrated within the path of liberation, we need to have a foundation. This foundation allows us to see and create change quickly. It allows hurts to arise, but more importantly, to go. What we let go of is our resistance. It is resistance that keeps us attached, keeps us limited, keeps us prideful and keeps us in pain. Resistance hides our emotions and then when they come out, still we cannot see them. When the charge becomes empty what is left is the great-perfection.

Muscles' shaking during a difficult exercise cleans the nerves, eliminates toxins, strengthens the will, and is a good meditation of being in the body. Judge your fitness with each exercise to avoid overly sore muscles; yet do not be afraid to get a few sore muscles here and there. We are applying ourselves for a larger effect than just muscle tone. We are putting pressure on our glands to secrete and open the inner spaces of our body to create and prepare the space of mediation.

Do not push through sharp pain or aggravation of an injury. In this case seek professional help, such as from a competent teacher.

If your muscles feel sore or tired after finishing a movement, it helps to slap them for fifteen to thirty seconds. Sometimes after an exercise such as horse stance, run in place for a minute and slap yourself all over at the same time in a silly rapid fashion. Slap the thighs, back, arms, chest, etc. It integrates the effects of the exercise in the body faster and feels wonderfully refreshing. Then sit or stand, and feel vitality at the navel, and keep the attention cognizant of the soft energy generated from the exercise permeating into the very bones and cells.

At the end of a Kriya and some exercises, a wonderful soft, alert and dissolved state is often experienced. Your chemistry is secreting various refined substances. Blockages to the deeper movement of our energy have been overcome. This is real nourishment. Stay with it for a while.

Some ABC's of the Yogic Path

Self-Empowerment Without the basis of self-responsibility, kriyas and practices never really bear fruit. Each must ultimately carry on their own shoulders responsibility for their peace, awakening, joy, understanding, mastery and beauty. Rather than blindly worshiping deities or constantly seeking the blessings of another, begin by becoming familiar with your own essence. A good place to start with is the feeling of your identity; what you look like, the feeling of recognition when someone calls your name, what it feels like to be centered deep inside of your body, and sensing your form, nonverbal awareness and style emanating forth as radiant light.

Refine, strengthen, and purify this awareness of your own aliveness. It is what you will always come back to. This is the means of staying awake as you penetrate into the inner realms. A sense of aliveness is what bridges the inner and outer. It is the call of clarity, and the elixir through which you will gather the forces of creation. In Eternal Yoga, we enter the Oneness through the characteristic of our individuality. Remember, definition equals wakefulness. Wakefulness equals awareness. As awareness is directed into the inner channels through practice, it becomes effortless self-radiance. Life becomes the ever-expanding perfection, when qualified as such.

Patience and Consistency Practice that which bears fruit. However, for any practice to bear fruit, our focus must become strong and unwavering. Gradually you will understand how to develop soft and turbulent free prana in the body and mind as an energetic support. Bring intention and attention by connecting to your depth to oversee and direct your outer-self. You are holding onto a subtle and at first inconsistent inner sense. It is like condensing mist into substance, slowly building a potency of connectivity upon which you can apply yourself. Sometimes resistance is slippery and crafty at distracting us from seeing blockages. You must learn to penetrate, and to develop the skill of directing your presence. Learn to distill and direct your breath as a subtle force. Learn to qualify that force with your own spark of aliveness, in different elemental ways. Over years of simple repetitive inner movement and focus we build a body out of enlightened presence.

Move Energy Do not become stagnant. If your thoughts or presence become scattered too much, or a practice becomes too mechanical, do something else to gain control of yourself. Be creative. Life includes everything; dancing, walking, relationship, sleeping… Learn to shift the perspective. Never let practices become a way of escaping life by keying out emotions and deeper issues. You can do techniques forever, yet without looking deeper into life, it will do little good in the long run. Always burn the candle from every end possible. Be physical, be formless, be consistent, be spontaneous, be invincible, be vulnerable - it is only in this way that you will gain the mastery to blend everything together as divine.

Intensity Give life your all. What is the point of simply being born, struggling, having a few experiences, dying and starting all over again and again and again? There has to be a certain realization of the preciousness of the moment, and a certain understanding not to settle for second best. To be wakeful is like being in Love. If you find it, without stabilizing it into greater undying awareness, is it not like meeting your beloved, then parting soon after? Intensity is not subject to the whims of social conformity, petty fears, and limitation. Be courageous, not fickle. Start with where you are at, and allow yourself to be seduced from within, day by day extending your inner penetration. Ignite bliss and mix it with everything; giving it a million nuances of what cannot be spoken. Grit, passion, presence; all these come from the intensity of a person who is deepening their essence. Decide what it is you really want! Then write it down and speak it often to yourself. Just how high and how deep are your spiritual goals?

A Progression of Practices

The approaches introduced in this book are:

- Burn the candle from every end possible (subtle and gross, formless and form, intensity and balance, inner and outer, self and relationship).
- You get there by being there.
- Consciously develop the continuum of your existence.

We begin to develop the continuum of our existence through grounding, connectivity and presence. Then we learn how to relax and expand within our presence. This is a general idea of how to progress through various practices in this series of books.

In the beginning, very defined techniques are the most helpful. Do not over-commit yourself, but do commit. What constitutes over-commitment is different for each person, but as a general guideline commit to a half-hour practice every day no matter what, and do the rest, even many hours of it, as part of your excitement. This is a practical approach that gets you through the tough spots and develops the all-important continuum. For those who are advanced, longer practice is necessary to penetrate into a deeper stabilization of reality. At this stage three or four hours most days is a minimum. As you advance, it is more the essence of what you are doing that is important, and you will use either rigid or fluidic forms of practice to develop that essence as appropriate.

Emotional work and re-imaging, clearing hurts, relationship ... is all interwoven with the techniques as part of our dynamic application. When you do not feel clear, do a practice, or do something to feel clear again. In that way you establish from the beginning what you are moving towards and you also create the positive habit of a yogi. There is a saying "more practice less drama, less practice, more drama." While (emotional) processing is important, if it is overdone, most people just keep on going in circles and start to thrive on the process of processing drama itself, instead of penetrating into deeper states of reality.

Music, dance, being in nature, service, ... you already understand according to your own inclinations and thus is not addressed here. There are souls who can achieve tremendous inner development from music. Just the same, I recommend expanding your possibilities with some of the wonderful gifts of the yogic disciplines.

I strongly suggest creating a yogic foundation emphasizing yogic-type individual practices. For those who aspire to the Tantric Path, I believe it is best to start on the Yogic path with Tantric overtones. As this matures over the years it develops into the Tantric path with Yogic undercurrents. I cannot emphasize the effectiveness of this approach enough.

On the following pages is a brief example of how a person can gradually progress through the three primary area of yogic practice addressed in this series of books. These three are preliminaries, eternal yoga and the tantras. Within each step you will have at different times a principle theme for a month, a year, or even a decade before the next step becomes workable. For example, within the preliminaries, it may take awhile just learning how to work with your body and breath, how to focus, etc. Then once you gain this, your application of various practices become more effective. At the right time your energy and motivation will naturally move you to further practices that now are in your reach, for example longer meditations, deeper penetrations, etc. Other examples of a theme may be greater awareness with a particular ray (such as blue or green ray for example) or element (such as fire or water), a relationship with a particular master, listening better, working principally within a particular chakra for awhile, developing greater compassion, etc. Each of these themes change in their overall depth as you advance, thus you may come back to a theme several times over the years.

You are getting your body and mind fit, flexible, soft, pliant, relaxed, delightful, and able to hold a focus without agitation. By all means explore the next steps, just understand that over time you will become much more able to effectively apply yourself at them. This foundation includes body-centered exercises and meditations, initial clearing and mastery of the energy flows within the body and initiatory openings of Eternal Yoga.

Step One – Create a Foundation through Preliminary Practices

Just Start	Even a little bit helps a lot.
Dynamic Yoga Sets. Meditate afterwards, as long as desired and you are not too sleepy or agitated. Create time for practice and become familiar with your self in quietude.	Vitality and openness helps to move through stuck energy and emotions. Your body, breath and mind all working together creates clarity, wholesomeness, radiance and an experience of the spiritual path.
Gradually refine your diet.	This will be somewhat automatic as you continue with your practice.
Add a Kriya Practice and deep, simple, aware, meditative breathing throughout your body (see simple breath kriya).	Moving the energy deeper inside and non-verbal development. Further clearing of energetic pathways and overcoming subtle levels of resistance. The simple breathing kriya is an “”essence”” practice, that over the years refines itself, opens you up, and develops your essence-nectar. Its fun!
Meditate early morning and before going to bed every day.	Now, this is becoming life!
Pay attention to your dreams, and try to remember them.	

Step Two – Awaken Into Your Primal Radiance with Eternal Yoga

Do the Eternal Yoga Practices.	Includes going above the head with integration into the body, awakening into buddhic awareness and initial development of an elemental vision of light. As introduced in "Tantra of the Beloved" and in more detail in the following book in this series.
Identify more with the Body of the One and intimately with one or more of the Ascended Masters.	Remain aware of your own presence. Develop insight and gain both transmission and reflection through this communion. Developing greater sensitivity to the greatest good. Do not get into channeling.

Step Three – Bring It All Together with the Fullness of Tantra

Create and center within your inner temple.	Includes a profound centering in one or more chakras and the central channel. Learning how to both absorb into and radiate out of the central channel. Non-dual awareness is very intimate.
Increase the nectars within your inner temple.	To give a home for your eternal light in the body. Relatively easy to do with proper foundation, almost impossible without it.
Profound integration.	Continuation of above, including consciousness 24 hours a day, dream yoga, sexual yoga if appropriate and greater levels of service.

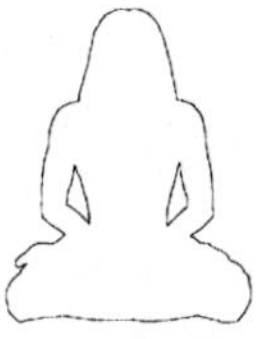

6

Locking and Containing Energy in the Body

Includes muscular and subtle energy locks, sitting positions and hand mudras.

Many body-orientated disciplines either consciously or instinctively use a contraction of various muscles to stimulate, contain and refine sexual essences and vital energy. These applications are known as *bhands* or locks. Secondary muscular coordination and connected visualization further circulates this energy and blends it with our mind-stream and the prana we breathe in.

In addition to the muscular locks, we also use *mudras,* which are circuits we create within our body or with another person so that energy flows within the specific pathways rather than escapes. Mudra translates as a "seal" or "sealing" of consciousness and energy, which results in the building of energy-substance to support a greater consciousness.

In the context of kriya practice, mudras are ways of holding our fingers, arms and posture to build energetic support for a particular type of composure or presence. Internal aspects include sensitivity to the circulation of energy through our channels.

In the tantras, mudra includes our state of consciousness in relation to others and our environment resulting in a non-dualistic way of viewing the world. Thus the Tantric application of mudra, by dissolving our limited perception and circulating energy and awareness in a greater context, frees our awareness into its true underlying radiant nature. It is a science that facilitates a building and blending of energy in an enlightened framework. Tantric mudra is covered in a later book in this series, as first we must create a foundation.

Our composure, whether sitting or engaging in dynamic movement, is of incredible importance in these practices and is reflective of our sincerity. The locks, mudras and proper sitting positions help us to connect with our subtle empowerment.

Mhula Bhanda and Associated Locks

Mhul means root. Thus mhula bhanda is a way of stimulating and directing energy from below the waist for use by the entire body. The application of this lock is one of the moist fundamental aspects of yoga, tantra and body orientated disciplines.

It consists of a coordinated contraction of the anus or perineum, the diaphragm at the base of the penis or the sides of the vagina, and to varying degrees the abdominal area. This is combined with a connected awareness of moving energy upwards, usually into the spine. The muscular contractions help to train or create a habit of how to move this energy, which as we progress becomes subtler and of a psychic nature. This results in the transformation of our essence-energy simply by connecting with it in an uplifting manner.

A light application of mhula bhanda naturally occurs during certain practices and when directing extra energy or calling upon extra energy. For example, when mediating at the third eye in connection with the whole body, this will create a natural increase of sexual energy[1], which because of our training in the locks, we instinctively draw upwards. Another example would be the automatic tightening of our muscles in a strenuous exercise to increase and bring up extra energy.

While mhula bhanda can be lightly applied with normal breathing, a stronger application is usually done with the breath held either in or out.

For an extra effect (with the breath held in) other muscles of the body are squeezed such as the legs, arms, chest, and buttocks in coordination with the primary locks. This generates additional vitality and clears our energy, lymph and blood. For more advanced practitioners, relying too much upon this extra help can detract from mastering the subtler and very important nuances of blending energy through finesse, where our energy flows upwards through the magnetic centering of our lifeforce.

To learn Mhula Bhanda, first do a few minutes of deep breathing and exercise to loosen up.

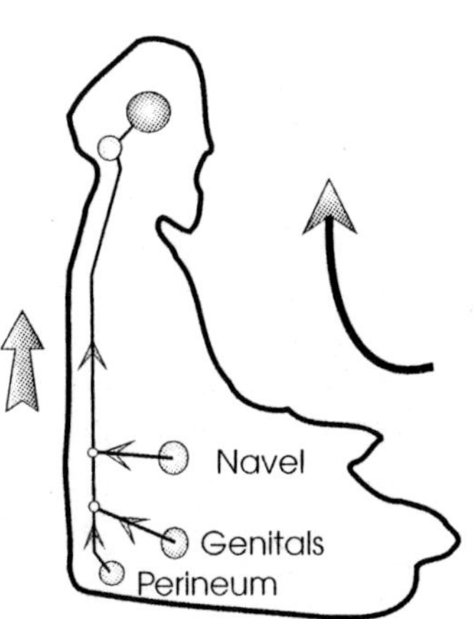

1 Sexual energy when refined is stored in the head. Correctly meditating in the head centers will cause an upward draw of sexual energy and an increase of vitality. As enough refined sexual substance collects in the brain, it first nourishes and vitalizes the brain, and then increases through the body to strengthen and nourish it. The cultivation and control of how refined sexual essence strengthens the physical and subtle body is a tantric art of the nectar body.

- Sit with a straight spine and bring attention to the perineum, which is located between the anus and the testicles or vagina. Inhale, hold the breath as long as comfortable, while contracting and releasing the perineum a few times, pulling it up on each contraction. For a mild contraction just the perineum is contracted. On a stronger contraction the buttocks, anus and testicles or vagina are also pulled up.

- Relax for a minute. Then inhale and hold, while contracting and relaxing the genitals a few times. Pull the genitals and the urogenital diaphragm up with each contraction. Relax between contractions.

- For the final component; inhale, hold and practice pulling the navel in towards the spine, feeling a connection from the navel to the spine and up the spine. Be sure that the neck is kept straight, the head slightly tucked back and the chin slightly tucked in. Alignment of the neck is extremely important. Be sure that the upper back is straight and relaxed, that is, do not arch the upper spine inwards. Energy may move directly into the spine, or else back down to the perineum and then up through the tailbone, or a combination. Gently squeeze the sides of the spine in an upward rippling fashion to direct energy up the spine into the lower part of the head. If the energy is cool and refreshing, it is fine to leave it in the head. If it is hot and expansive, then be sure to bring it back down the front to the navel area. This is often down after the lock, with a normal breath and a sense of tingling ease flowing down the body.

- Bring all the components together into one smooth movement. Inhale, hold and pull in the genitals, then the perineum a fraction of a second later, and then joined by pulling the navel into towards the spine, bringing the combined momentum up the spine. Hold for the duration of the breath, as comfortable. Practice at first with the breath held either in or out. In time, you should feel a fullness of energy in the lower centers and the spine. You want to develop a continual subtle-magnetic coupling of the energy from your root centers into the command of the navel region, so as to create a flow of nourishing upward energy.

As you pull up the perineum, direct the warm energy into the base of the spine and up the spine. Pulling in the navel further enhances the effect and keeps the energy in the spine, rather than floating out to the front of the body. Contract the muscles along the sides of the spine in rhythm with the upward movement of attention into the head. These contractions help you feel your spine, intensify the energy and keep it contained on its path.

If the energy is allowed to travel on the back of the spine, towards the skin, then the energy may be too hot when it arrives in the head, creating dizziness. When I talk about bringing energy up the spine, I am referring to the spinal marrow, which is several inches inwards from the skin. In this way, when the energy arrives into the head, it will be refreshing, expansive and grounding at the same time, and feel like a tonic.

When practicing with the breath held in, the navel should not feel empty after you finish exhaling. Rather you should leave some of the energy in the navel, somewhat like a continually lit fire. In this way the energy builds better and you will have much more control of it (note: you should physically exhale all the breath out).

As a variation you can hold the breath and bring the energy only up to the navel region, more towards the back than the front, then as you exhale, keep it mostly at the navel chakra, feeling it being absorbed there. It is important to distinguish the difference between the belly-button and the navel chakra. The navel point or belly button is on your frontal line, while the navel chakra is deep in the body towards the spine. When inhaling, be sure to breath down into the lower abdomen, so that the downward movement of the incoming prana, contains the upwards movement of the locks at the navel, mixing with it. You are pushing down the energy of your breath and pulling up the earthiness of your root. When done correctly you will not feel dizzy. This variation is the basis of vase breathing which is presented more fully in the section on inner fire practice.

Mhula bhanda creates countless benefits, including vitality, a strong heart and a light vibrant feeling in the head. If the lower centers feel drained or weak, mhula bhanda will help to rebuild your presence in this area. If there is an abundance of energy, it directs that energy upwards, helping to transmute it in the process, so that it does not become an agitation.

Mhula bhanda is both a physical and a psychic lock that trains you to recognize the pathway of transmutation. Contracting the muscles is simultaneously accompanied by a mental visualization and intention, which greatly enhances the whole effect. In fact, as the pathway becomes clear and second nature, the power of thought alone keeps a constant upward pleasant-feeling force in action, wiring the control centers in your head to the lower centers. Without this wiring, the body is not able to move in total harmony with the higher intentions of your spirit.

This lock can be used in many applications, such as martial arts, yoga, and sports, even walking down the street with a contained energy. You do not always have to hold the breath in or out while applying this lock, although for an intense application, it helps. A martial arts stance, such as horse stance, is a great way to get really familiar with mhula bhanda.

As the lock becomes familiar, you will understand how to modify its components suitably. For example, in some yoga poses it may be more appropriate to apply a stronger navel lock, in others only a slight tension at the navel. In advanced practices, where a moist and intense inner fire is built by drawing in all of our lifeforce at or just below the level of the navel, towards the spine, the very subtle and deep flow of energy is the most important aspect paid attention to. In this practice, our outer prana is brought into the sphere of our inner radiance and infused with it to enlighten the whole body. The practice becomes effortless and very blissful, if properly done. However, if this practice if forced before we are ready, then all we end up creating is a willful fire, anger, and bodily disorders. Yogic practice cannot be intellectually and ambitiously forced in an egotistical sense, rather, through the intensity of our commitment to the bigger picture, we refine and make transparent the crystal of our being over years, and thus remain natural, wholesome, and become liberated right where we stand.

A woman on her moon cycle, or in the later stages of pregnancy, should not apply mhula bhanda.

An Energy Tonic through the Art of Containment

At the end of a chant or breathing exercise, it is often recommended to hold the breath as long as comfortable. For beginners this may only be twenty seconds, but as you gain experience this can become a minute or longer. The energy may increase much more rapidly than you anticipate. Thus it is extremely important to have a straight spine, neck lock and a strong navel lock; keep the energy contained. Of primary importance is your focus of attention in the body. Do not space out or let your mind wander into thoughts. If you are loosing it, do not exhale until you have regained control of the energy. Otherwise the rising energy will shoot off into space or through a minor channel and create heat in the brain. You will most likely get dizzy and even blackout. If energy travels up the spine correctly, but the neck is not held properly, then it can generate a force that may throw you several feet. It has happened to me a number of times, such as being tired from getting home late at night, practicing a mild kriya such as Sa-Ta-Na-Ma, not much really occurring, I hold my breath carelessly, and.... Other times it has occurred in moments of letting my mind wander during a pranayama.

To help gain control of energy that might overwhelm you, immediately squeeze the muscles of the neck and large muscles of the body while inwardly pressing down into your navel chakra and pulling up the anus. When the energy builds and you contain it, it creates a wonderful clarity and health benefit. You feel on top of the world.

Any time you create a soft prana in the body, such as through meditation, pranayama, or visualization, it is beneficial to end the practice by tightening the muscles of your body. Isolating different muscles in a wave like movement. This drives energy deeper into the bone marrow. While squeezing the muscles, mhula bhanda will be automatic. It is important that you simultaneously visualize and feel soft energy moving into your bones and waking you up. As the breath is not held, there is no danger in this practice of misalignment. Rather, at times it brings to the forefront a feeling similar to making love, whereby you squeeze a few muscles and feel exhilarated in the containment. Finish by relaxing for a few minutes while absorbing the energy. This can also be done in the middle of a session to keep contained and for refreshment. If you have to go somewhere right after a kriya session, do some of the contractions and visualizations as you get up and get yourself ready. Add a skip in your step, perhaps a minute of horse stance; feel good. In advanced tantric stages, these contractions are only occasional necessary because the energy is already deep and integrated in the body.

Squeezing and relaxing the anus is a wonderful health tonic, which can give you extra strength to fend off a cold or to keep going when you are tired. Inhale and hold the breath for a few seconds while squeezing the anus and then relax the breath and the anus. Practice so that you can feel yourself squeezing tightly and several inches up into the rectum. While exhaling gently direct a sense of vitality up through the tailbone and lower spine. Through consistent practice you will gradually gain a better connectivity that allows you to direct energy with your mind alone or in combination with the breath.

Meditative Sitting Positions

In regards to formal sitting positions, the best is to triangulate the body so as to give a stable position with a straight spine in which it is easy to be still. Sitting on a chair works for shorter sittings (up to a half hour), but not so well for longer times. Sitting on the floor or ground with crossed legs such as in the following positions of easy pose, half-lotus and full lotus are suitable. Sore knees work themselves out over time, especially if we are exercising, have a reasonable diet, and know how to, or are learning how to, work with our sexual energy in a fulfilling and regenerating way. A firm cushion such as a futon or a sheepskin is helpful; however sitting on a soft mattress is a hindrance.

Obviously, if there is a lot of difficulty in a formal sitting position, do the best you can. Assistance can really help at this time. For example, a teacher may have you do a certain practice lying in bed combined with other practices of sitting in a chair and perhaps addressing other areas of your life. Never feel that you cannot start from whatever condition you presently are in.

When engaging in silent practice, it is fine to shift leg positions several times during the course of a sitting and to stretch a bit here or there. In a chanting kriya or pranayama it is better to try and maintain an unmoving position or else a very integrated movement that is part of the building presence. The reason for the difference has to do with the method in which potency builds. Kriya-chants and pranayama require an unbroken building of particular kinds of prana in the body so as to absorb the monkey-mind and enter non-conceptual reality. This occurs in a very powerful manner. In contrast, in silent practice we simply hold our attention in a particular mode or place within the body, and our thought and energy shifts into the natural quality of that mode or place. If we stretch here or there, it does not have to effect this alignment and the freshening effect often helps us. The only reason we are staying still is to aid the firm placement of our attention and to transfer some of our vitality into a subtle vehicle. In time this attention can be and should be held within the dynamic quality of movement.

In silent practice we are either attempting to enter a depth, or are already in that depth and expanding within it. Once we are in this second phase sitting still is effortless, as our attention and energy has become absorbed into the central core of our body. By sitting with a straight spine it is easier to bring our attention and energy into our core, which is a requirement for entering our depth. In fact just sitting in a proper meditation position alone can bring us into meditation by helping us to maintain wakefulness as we go within. If we loose our inner bearings, i.e., if we are not centered within one of the chakras or channels, we loose the energetic support for staying awake and our meditation goes nowhere. Starting out with formal kriyas is wise, because of kriyas potency in facilitating this grounding.

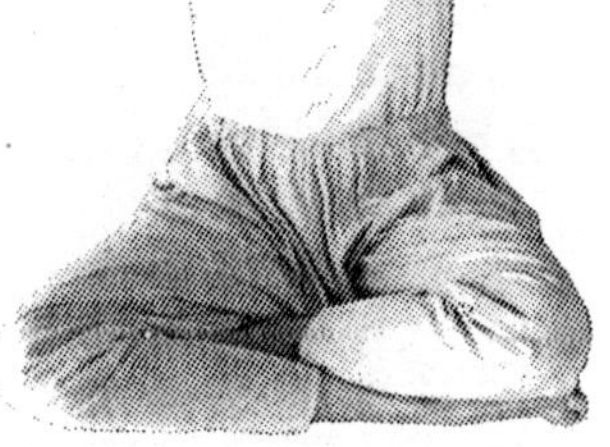

Easy pose is sitting with our legs crossed in the most comfortable way (this is my favorite).

In **Lotus pose**, we cross the legs so each foot rests on top of the opposite thigh. This can take some getting use to and perhaps several months or a few years for it to be easy. Lotus pose helps to keep the lower back locked straight so that it does not slump in the course of our practice. This includes keeping our tailbone straight so that vitality moves

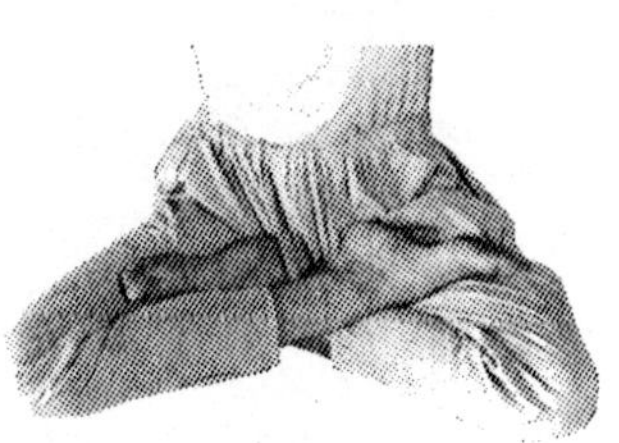

into it and up our spine. When energy flows through our tailbone, everything is easier, lighter, and energetic. We are more secure in ourselves and thus able to relax beyond grasping which is one of the definitions of meditation.

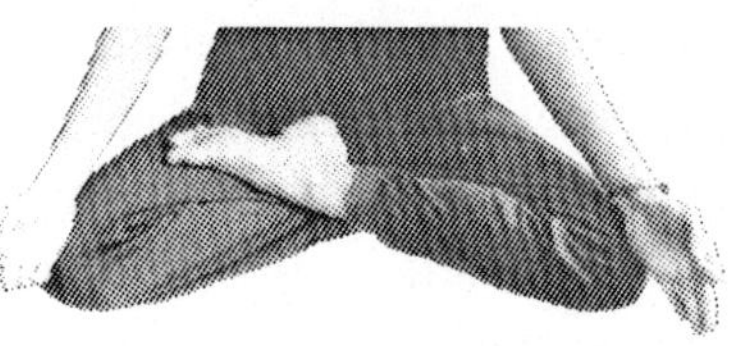

Half-Lotus is an alternative where we place only one foot at a time on the opposite thigh. (My next favorite sitting position.)

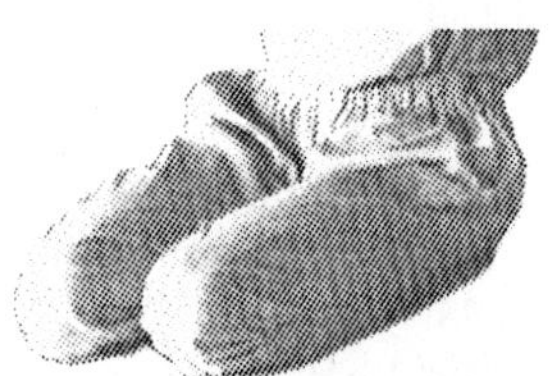

Sitting on the heels stimulates digestion and is sometimes used for variety and by some kriyas. A variation is sitting between the heals, which is also called celibate pose.

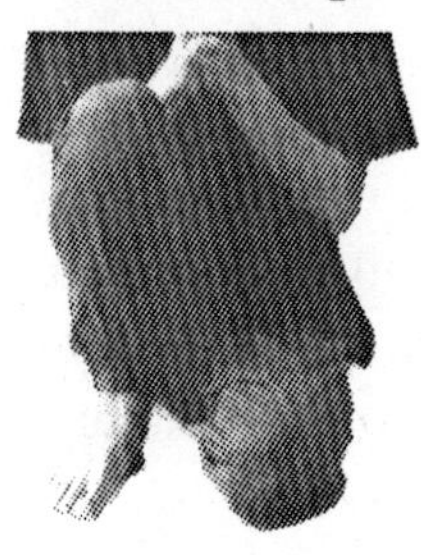

Warrior pose is sitting on one heal with the other foot flat on the ground. It is called this because a warrior could rise quickly from sitting to standing if the need arose. It creates an alert energy and is used by some of the kriyas. A variation used for variety when sitting and as a stretch is to place the foot flat on the ground on the other side of the knee, commonly with the hands resting on the upright knee.

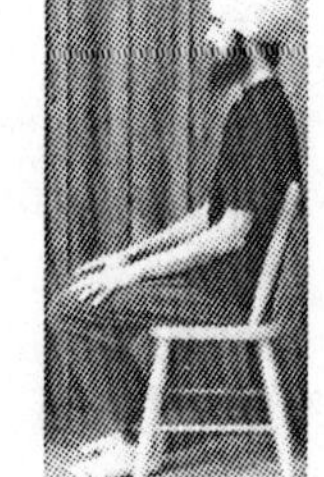

For those wanting or needing to **sit on a chair**, sit with both feet flat on the ground and the back straight.

As the lower back becomes strong and open, then it becomes easy to sit with the legs in many different ways for variety, such as stretched out or wide apart. Pictures of Tara with one leg stretched out is an example.

While sitting there should be a kind of sexual potency below the navel that is drawn up to the navel area and into the body. This kindles our moist-inner fire or energetic aliveness. This potency happens automatically in response to the upper centers opening up, unless we disassociate with the body. This potency is further kindled and contained by lightly contracting the anus upwards.

Occasionally you will automatically contract these muscles strongly and you can feel several inches up into the rectum. If the lower back slumps backwards or is held too far forward, then this potency does not accumulate because the tailbone does not open up and the kidneys do not come into play. If you lean too far forwards, or if you try to pull the lower back in too much, it tends to shut the back of the heart down. This prevents an open-expansive feeling and keeps energy locked up into the head. By resting the hands on the knees and perhaps leaning back very slightly while gently expanding the upper back out (a slight outward bow), remembering to keep the lower back and tailbone straight, will correct this. Keep the shoulders relaxed (sunk) down. The neck should be straight and locked slightly back so that the big vertebrae in the back of the neck comes in. Tuck the chin slightly down. Proper alignment of the neck is extremely important for mixing energy in the body. By opening the eyes slightly and looking down past the tip of the nose, you balance the two sides of your body and maintain a better spatial firmness of attention within your body (so you do not space out). Everything floats in balance. You are relaxed and wakeful, poised and fresh, neither stiff nor slumped.

A benefit of crossing the legs to meditate is that this lessons the flow of energy to the legs, and thereby increases the amount of energy available for an upward circulation. Notice the word lessens, not eliminate. There should be some flow of energy to the legs.

Hand Mudras

The first two hand mudras in the following list are the most common. Many more hand mudras are given later in the book that are specific to various kriya practices.

- **Gyan mudra.** First finger and thumb tips joined together with hand resting on knees. Calming effect on the mind that is integrated with the breath. A variation is for the finger to curl up slightly under the thumb, so the tip touches the crease between the segments of the thumb.

- **Buddha mudra.** Hands resting in lap, palms up, one hand on top of the other with the thumb tips touching. Generally, men place the right hand on top and ladies the left hand on top. Good for when we forget about the breath and move into our inner vibrant core. The thumb tips touching helps to neutralize our outward movement of attention.

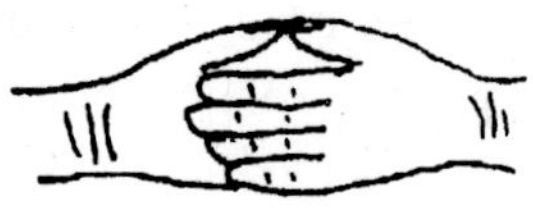

- **Vajra fists.** The method given here is a variation popularized in a number of practices within Tibetan Buddhism. The thumb touches the first or second inside joint of the ring (sun) finger. The fingers close over the thumbs into loose fists. The hands rest on the knees palms down. This method is good for internalizing our energy, particularly for kindling the inner fire at the navel. It develops a sensual coziness. When meditating for some time with the hands in this mudra, when you finish take a few minutes to relax and notice your surroundings before opening the hands and releasing the thumb.

- **Prayer mudra.** The palms of the hands are joined, as in prayer, with the base of the hands from the bottom of the thumbs to the wrist touching the chest, between the nipples. This is very centering and calming, as it balances the two sides of our body, our masculine and feminine aspects, at the heart center. Particularly good to integrate and balance after an intense set or pranayama. Also as the name suggest, it is good for prayer. A variation is to lower the forehead to the ground while keeping the hands in prayer mudra. This variation enlivens a sense of innocence and is very healing.

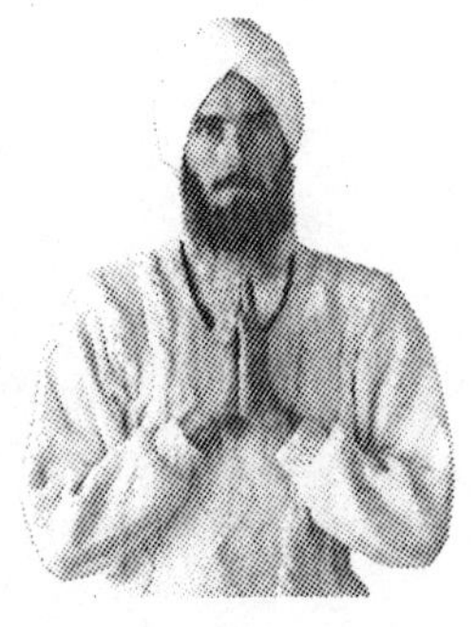

- **Gracefully moving arms and hands like in a dance.** Once we are established within our nonverbal movement of energy within the body, this is incredibly wonderful and alive.

Sitting straight in full lotus, anus pulled up slightly and abdomen pulled in slightly, upper back not contracted inwards, neck lightly locked and chin tucked. Eyes part way open looking down past the tip of the nose, hands either in the lap on Buddha Mudra of resting on the knees, such as in Vajra Fist method of holding the thumbs inside the fists; these collectively are known as the seven-points of Vairochana's meditation posture (a Buddhist master from the time of Padmasambhava). In the Buddhist tradition these seven-points are widely taught and attention is traditionally given to perfecting them.

In contrast there are very advanced tenants of practice that advocate whatever position we happen to be in as our meditation posture. Of course this natural approach is the best, provided we have the corresponding capacity. You may have some of your best meditations lying in bed, slouched on a couch, doing some activity, or whatever. Yet, for the sake of consistency and practicality, practice in formal ways as your daily mainstay.

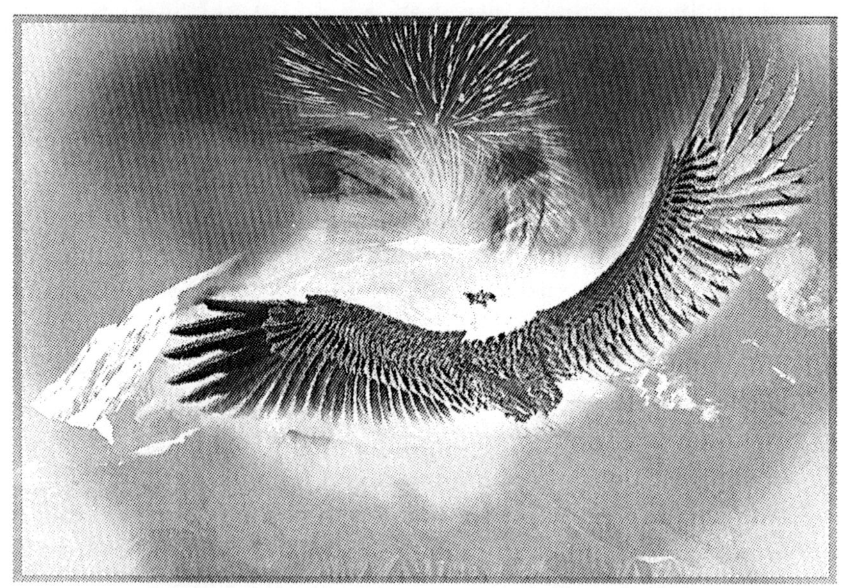

I have found that the secret of spiritual development lies in the body ....

The physical is but the outer show of a vast play, incomprehensible, yet very intimate...

Discover what this body is!

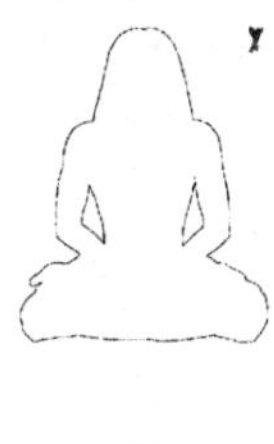

7

The Magic of Breathing

Skilled and conscious breathing is at the very heart of the yogic way. Conscious breathing enables us to increase and direct energy into greater awareness, grounding and joy. By intimately understanding the inseparable relationship of consciousness and energy, we awaken and enliven desirable qualities, such as radiance, increased compassion, bliss, strength, and penetrating insight. By understanding that the body is energy, we enhance and create our body to play in the energy dance of our greater beingness.

To realize the potential of our breath we must merge gross and subtle breathing together. Learning how to breathe easily, fully, and correctly is an important first step. Exercise, stretching, diet, emotions and health all affect the ability to breathe easily.

The keys to activate our subtle breath are connectivity, visualization and feeling, all of which are enhanced through meditative practice. The various breathing techniques and kriyas given in this book provide an opportunity to practice this melding of the physical and subtle breath. By bringing our prana deeper and more grounded within ourselves, we are supporting a deeper and more restful state of awareness and our chitchat mind naturally becomes silent. In this potency of silence we gain inner reflection and become more familiar with ourselves. This familiarity brings connectivity, by which we can start to become masters of ourselves. Connectivity, visualization, and abiding in our visualization so as to gain substance allow us to generate and collect the inner nectars and thus embrace the inner tantras. All of this starts with the magic of breathing.

The natural and proper way to breathe is to drop the diaphragm down as we inhale. The navel, sides and kidney area will all expand out, which in turn pulls the diaphragm down, thus inflating the lungs. At times when we want an extra big inhale, we will finish the inhale by filling out the upper lungs, i.e., the upper chest as well. By primarily using the navel area to inhale, we better assimilated the energy of our breath and can more easily direct it. This movement circulates our spinal fluids, relaxes the heart, gives us strength, and helps to distill energy from the breath.

In this way we slow down the breath while making it fuller and deeper. By slowing down the breath everything becomes more connected, less rushed, and we have a better sense of direction in our life. A whole body sense is created. Rubbing the sides of your ribs at the level of the solar plexus helps to open up the breath.

As we clear out congestion our breathing becomes both effortless and full. During some of the yoga exercises, we can breath in an exaggerated manner, i.e., taking in more air than we actually need. The extra breath will be distilled into soft energy that the body can handle in unlimited quantities. However, if your feel dizzy, slow down or stop; do not push yourself into further dizziness. There should be an effortless quality to deep breathing. It takes time for this clearing, and our ability can vary from one day to the next. It is also important that there is a feeling of "substance" inside the body with which the breath can combine. This substance is the potency of yin fluids in the body, which takes time to build. Without this, the extra energy is not held and contained in a constructive manner, which can lead to headaches, feeling up and down - energetic one moment and then lifeless the next. A proper diet and tonic herbs can help this tremendously Also it takes time to learn how to digest the extra energy.

By remaining present and cultivating a rich feeling inside the body while breathing deeply, there is easily ten times the benefit to the dynamic yoga exercises. It all works together, the deep breathing gives you more energy to be present, which you are moving and deepening through the exercise, which gives you more capacity. This combination assumes that you are also connecting to the soft and cosmic aspects of your breath, through presence. This occurs as we become more in our bodies both in a physical spatial sense and an energetic sense. Until this connectivity is gained, vary your approach. Sometimes breathe deeply, sometimes softly. When you breathe deeply feel yourself blasting through. When you breathe softly, it is not air, but a very fine prana, connectivity itself that you are breathing. Eventually you will bring the two together.

The cosmic soft breath can be so enriching, awakening, expansive and nourishing that at times it is appropriate to forget about the physical breath altogether, so as to better be present with it.

As the body becomes more vitalized and the outer channels cleared of agitation, then a subtle breath may be engaged in, where the physical breath is ignored or forgotten about. This occurs deep within the body. This breath is not necessarily the in and out motion of the physical breath, rather, it is the flow of subtle radiance, sometimes directed through the vibratory focus of mantra and sometimes through simple natural awareness. It is a deep internalizing of our attention.

A good way to develop the cosmic breath is to visualize yourself radiant in light originating from the core of your body, magnetically drawing in and radiating out a substance of light and ecstasy. It may work better for you to make the actual place(s) of bright radiance small in size, and then let the rest of the body become lit up from it. You attention does not wander from this, and your outer breath helps to further ignite the potency of this cosmic breath, yet remains secondary to it. Vast fluidic worlds of ecstatic consciousness will open within you over the years.

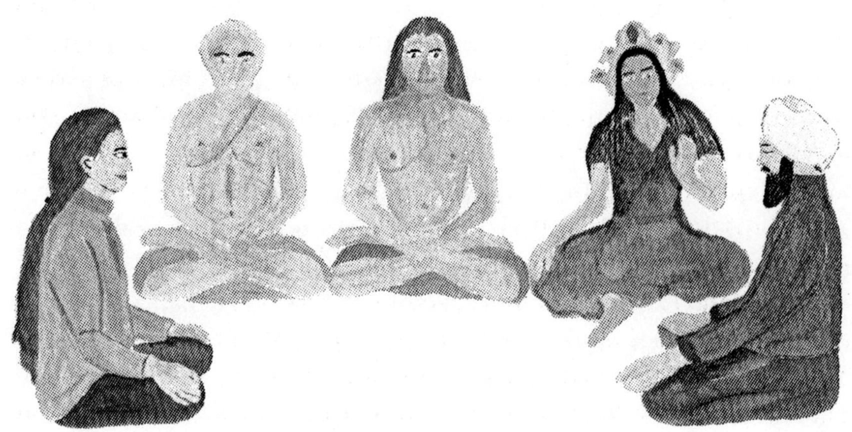

An Everyday Kriya of Simple Breath

Each and everyday sit quietly and begin to breathe slow and deep. As you become more internalized, do not stop the breath, but continue. Do this at least five or ten minutes and preferably for 30 minutes to an hour. However do not time it with a watch.

As you breathe, connect your breath to become a source of vitality. While breathing down into your belly, direct the energy form the breath through an organ, or up and down your spine, or through your hands for example. Be sure, that as you connect with an area you keep the energy soft and open, while making the focus more and more precise. Without this soft open feeling the extra energy can result in congestion.

As you inhale feel that you are drawing energy into the body and as you exhale keep the energy in the body. On the exhale, concentrate the breath and attention together so that you can feel its subtle movement. While deep full breathing is important, it is more important that you connect with the subtlety of the breath. When this connection is present it becomes easy for the breath to be both deep and slow (approximately two to four times per minute). This should not be forced; rather cultivate over time. Do not try and force your breathing to be super deep, rather just make it as deep as is comfortable and natural.

Make sure to connect to the tan tien (just below the navel and in) and then expand to other areas of the body. Some days you may use a whole sitting focusing just on your tailbone area, or your liver, or within the heart, or the third eye, or the spine, etc. Another day you may move around much more. Give yourself the freedom to penetrate into the inner spaces and the space of every place.

Do not breath directly into the heart area for more than a few minutes and make sure you are first bringing the bulk of the breath into your navel area. The heart requires a very delicate balance of energy, which the body creates all by itself. Focusing too much physical energy into the heart can cause it too miss beats or become painful. If this occurs, focus down into your navel, brush the energy down your chest with your hands, have a glass of water, and stop the practice. Go for a walk, or take a nap to balance out. When you are experienced in practice (over the years) and gradually learn how to penetrate into the heart center, then you can coordinate this with the breath as following. Your energy rises from below and energy from your head sinks down into a common meeting point. This is a precision affair and the points of entry are small, perhaps a quarter inch in size. This is located between the nipples and slightly more towards the back than the front. However the results are big, as a subtle radiance deep within the heart opens up your whole life and perspective. The breath is anchored in the tan tien area and some of its energy transfers through this point of juncture in the heart and further opens up the chest. The breath fans the energy available to rise from below and sink from above.

While the primary way of enhancing awareness of the breath having substance is through paying attention to its effects as it moves through a part of your body, also at times work with sensations of density, emptiness, color, warmth, coolness, or presence. Feel your blood, your sexual juices, inside your bones, your face, and your inner spaces. Be sure to keep the focus inside your body. Cultivate awareness of a whole-body feeling.

There is really no limit to this simple and natural way of meditating. No dharma or organization can claim it. You are so obviously free, that you can do real meditation on the spark of your existence. Learn to breathe your spirit and experience what this means. Continue to breathe deeply until you feel really alive. Then breathe that radiant image into your tissues, that they become the flesh of spirit. Learn to concentrate (not dissipate) the subtlety of breath and the nectars that follow.

There are a thousand variations, such as exhaling toxins out, inhaling light in, exhaling heaviness out, inhaling ease in, exhaling light out, exhaling light in, swimming in the cosmic ocean. You may also guide the energy of your breath through one of the principal energy routes, such as the microcosmic orbit (described later in the book).

Learning to concentrate and contain the energy received from subtle breath is a vital key to this practice. Generally in the beginning you inhale energy in and exhale it out. This is fine for initial purification, but should naturally change to a different approach as will be described. Subtle energy and connectivity is inhaled into the body and into the bones. During the exhale your energy is contained and built upon, or when of sufficient force it is moved through routes "within" the body. While exhaling, do not loose touch with the presence of energy already inhaled. Thus the feeling is that with each inhale you add to the energy and with each exhale it becomes more tangible in the body. A continuity develops that is beyond the in and out of the breath. Using the navel area to regulate your energy becomes extremely important so that not too much prana is built up in sensitive areas, such as your heart, before it is refined and the channels are opened more.

Everything in this practice is experiential. Do not jump ahead of this. For example, first build and feel within one area such as your hands, before trying some larger area. There is no shortcut, although you can accelerate the process under guidance by adding additional supportive practices. Over the months you will feel lighter, with a greater spring in your step, and a natural support to understand the transparent nature of reality. Rather than exhaling energy out of the body, you will start to glow. This radiance is less fickle in nature, because it emanates from a deeper place in your body.

With the breath you learn to mix your mind with your emotional and sexual energy. The steadiness and direction of your mind directs the breath, which becomes enlivened with your emotional substance. In this way you are drawing your own self into your inner temple, whereby you can experience enlightenment. Sexual life force gives us greater tangibility. This movement refines the sexual life force into nectar throughout the body that supports greater consciousness.

As you clear the mind and refine sexual energy you will naturally value maintaining sexual potency. With your mind you bring the sexual energy into the bone marrow, which is regenerating. There will at times be an instinctual pulling up of and refining of your sexual energy through mhula bhand. This inward turning of your sexual life force may at first lesson your sexual desire because the energy is being used to fill the inner reservoirs. This is a good sign. Latter, it will come forth again in increased drive. Your mind grows into spirit and is thus transformed from a common mentality into a rich, vibrant, juicy, radiant expansive wholesomeness.

After you have built a foundation within your physical body, grow your energy presence to include the area above your head and below your feet. Go into the chakras, channels and nectars. Ignite the male and female making love and bring it into the innermost core of your body. Prepare the birthing ground of spirit into immortal form.

Practice being aware that, your senses and what they sense, exists inside of your self. Hear all sounds as a singing of existence. Breathe naturally and deeply into the body and become aware of the breath originating within the top of the head, not in a sense of just breathing through the top of the head, but "originating" from the top of the head as the beautiful soul our body resides within. This is indescribable, yet to breath is something we all do. Do not settle for quiescence too quickly by letting the breath go and fleeing into breathless tranquility. Rather merge the two together to penetrate and integrate.

Awaken to that silent breathless presence, by focusing in on it. But then hearken it to every cell, by the physical and subtle breath. Thus you will simultaneously work with a still radiant energy that does not oscillate with the in and out energy of the breath. Enliven your tissues to receive the very subtle still light. Feel the aliveness of your internal image, which from a physical viewpoint, lives on faint airs, yet has the power to direct, shape, and become the physical state of being. This ignites bliss, regeneration, beauty and more.

In purifying, bringing out, getting in touch with and refining your own presence, you will be able to better commune with the presence of others and as a result widen you own identity. Wonderful is the Oneness!

Be happy for no reason at all. Be free in yourself and let the world reflect into that. Embrace life, relationship, and become fearless of any fear in applying yourself and gaining your own mastery. What a great present to give yourself and everyone you touch.

Make this kriya a practice you do everyday, no matter what else. Some days it may be for an hour or more, other times a few minutes as a kind of internal warm up. Do other practices so you can do this practice better and this practice so you can do other practices better. The benefits will be immeasurable.

May all beings be blessed and bless all beings.

Skin, Bone and Organ Breathing

This area is seldom given the attention it deserves in many traditions, and through this lack of attention there is sometimes giving the impression that this type of further grounding into the body is not necessary. To the contrary, we have received direct advise of the importance of this grounding from some of the most developed masters on this planet who have demonstrated an eternal existence projected into the physical for a long time.

The Cosmic Masters Meru and Mu [1] talk to us of the soul within each organ and how that must be developed and grounded to create a regenerating body. It is a wonderful practice to feel an organ as consciousness. To do so requires focused attention within our body and the nurturing of the subtle essences or nectars in each part of the body. This type of practice becomes quickly integrated with other practices such as dynamic yoga, meditation and the tantras.

This type of practice is very natural, because it uses, without unnecessary contrivance, your already existing body and its wisdom, your breath, creativity and awareness. A person of sensitivity who is doing the inner work, even if they had never received instruction of this kind could naturally end up doing this kind of activity.

Grounding into and the energetic refinement of the organs and tissues of the body are a much-needed support for tantric development. When directing the energy of the breath into an organ or tissue, keep the awareness there soft and open. Following are meditations on breathing through tissues, bones, organs and the skin.

Bone Breathing

This is a fantastic, easy to do, and very beneficial practice. It is easily adaptable to various situations such as proper sitting, lying in bed, while driving (being careful to maintain full presence), for a person confined to bed, to move past a stuck feeling, to internalize your mind, etc...

1 Mu is also known as VajraYogini or Vajra Vairochani. Meru is also known as Garab Dorje

Bone breathing is simply absorbing and circulating subtle energy into and through our bone marrow. This can be done with or without coordination with the physical breath.

Bones are living, breathing and vibrating crystals upon which we imprint our deepest physical memories, instincts, hopes and fears. Inside our bones is marrow, which includes our brain. Do not think of bones like a picture of a dead skeleton; rather reflect on them as living tissues. Bone marrow stores the body's reserves and is created out of a combination of refined sexual essences, blood and fat. By breathing through our bones we direct extra sexual energy into them, which makes us light and vibrant. In the process, we burn out congestion and unnecessary fat.

Obtaining awareness within our bones gives us connectivity and grounding. When we move a leg, we feel the spatial quality of that leg, the location of that leg, and the bones within our leg. With our eyes closed we still have a very connected effortless energetic picture of our leg in relation to our environment. We are pervaded by an inner calmness and security that is always present.

There exist whole spiritual disciplines based around cleansing and elevating our bone marrow and tendons, such as those introduced by Bodhidharma to the Shaolin monks. These practices are not just for health but to attain enlightenment.

There are two general approaches to bone breathing. The first and easiest is to start with the feet or hands and to breath energy into them, gradually going through the bone structure deep into the body. The second approach is to first cultivate an energy source, usually in the lower abdomen and then lead this into the bone marrow, such as through the tailbone and into the ribs, gradually cleansing and elevating the bone marrow of the entire body. As the practice progresses, extra sexual energy is stimulated, yet contained, which becomes nectar within our bones that supports the continuum of awareness of our very subtle, our subtle and our physical existence.

The second practice is quite advances in all the details of cultivation and thus best learned through an instructor. However in a less intense form this is good to combine with the first approach. For example, breath for awhile into the lower abdomen and build up energy there. Then switch to slowly breathing in energy through the hands for example. The energy from your lower abdomen helps your concentration and it brings substance, such as your sexual substances into the blood to combine with the energy you are breathing in through your hands. Also by first building up an energy at the lower abdomen, it will be easier to breath the energy through the bones from a hand or foot, into the arm or leg bones, and from there into the spinal marrow.

When breathing through the finger or toes, feel inside of your thumbs or your big toes while breathing through them. In this connectivity, you will eventually feel the spatial quality, the joints will creak and a tingling will be felt. Continuing to use the breath, inhale energy in. At first you may exhale the energy back out, but after awhile you should contain the energy while exhaling. While inhaling further energy in, do not loose connectivity with the energy already present from the previous exhale. In this way the energy builds.

As you build an energy presence and lightness, gradually inhale through more of your bones. For example, we inhale energy through all of our toes, then through the bones of our feet and into our ankles. We may spend many sessions just getting energy built up into and clear within our ankles. It is amazing how much energy our joints can contain. Anyone who has sprained an ankle will attest to this. In fact, the fluids within our joints is in some yogas called a second semen, because of the quality and quantity of electrically refined energy and essence this fluid can contain.

As marrow becomes cleared of fat and toxins, in future sessions, it is quickly charged and thus we progress to the next set of bones. Generally, work through the legs up to the lower spine. Then we work through the hand and arms into the shoulders, scapula, spine and ribs. You can intermix the legs and arms from one session to the next or even work on both simultaneously. Then we combine the energy from the legs and arms in the spine in the area opposite of the solar plexus. From here we move back up the spinal marrow into the back of the head. The back of the head stores refined essence, which in turn opens the third eye. As the head fills with nectar, it drips back down into the body where it is absorbed, or circulated back up. This nectar tastes like honey. Do not be in a rush; think months or years.

There are variations on the above theme that will present themselves to you. For example, at times you may bring energy from the legs and lower body directly up the spine into the head without further mixing. At times you may use only your mind to bring in and direct energy (instead of the breath and mind). At times you may use neither the breath nor the mind, but simply the emotional richness of your being penetrating through your bones. You may bring energy in through different routes simultaneously. You may draw in energy from other places besides the feet and hands, including direct origination from the etheric centers.

Tissue and Organ Breathing

This is a whole path in itself; in which you cultivate and collect various energies in each organ and then blend these energies. Details are only touched upon here. For many this is sufficient, however for those needing detailed maps much more information is available in various Taoist practice books.

Each organ supplies the type of energy necessary to support particular emotions. When purified and harnessed, vibrant organ energy can be used to generate refined emotions that are of tremendous value on the tantric path, particularly in creating a body of nectar.

Each organ has a primary characteristic of energy and emotion that it supports. In organ breathing we simply direct a quality of energy into an organ. This flushes the organ of toxins and brings up stored emotions, memories, and vitality within the organ. As this occurs, the increased flow of energy-substance through the organ improves aspects of our awareness and health.

Filling the kidneys with energy increases our sense of presence. We become calmer, stronger and surer of ourselves, which allows a gentle, helpful nature to come forth. Our sexual vitality, bone marrow and reserves our all intimately connected with the kidneys. The kidneys support courage and intimacy. It is important to keep the kidneys strong, for this gives us resilience. Some healing systems call the kidneys the hospital of the body. When you enter the soul of your kidneys you enter into a very deep mystical aspect of yourself whereby you can recreate yourself. Colors often associated with the kidneys are blue and white along with a watery quality. Sometimes red has a place to warm the kidneys.

The liver is a huge organ, which makes it easy to focus energy within it. It is under your ribs on the right side of the body. A green color works nicely. Sometimes a deep red has its place in the liver. Feel the liver as smooth in texture and harmonious in nature. The liver gives us warmth and visual acuity. It is often one of the most emotional of the organs to cleanse, and an out of balance liver gives impulsiveness and anger. The liver stores images of our self. Place you hand on it to help connect with it. Feel its ability to purify the body. The liver stores soul experience and the images that this evokes, including images of what we think we can or cannot do, or who we feel we are. It gives us drive and sometimes agitation. Much of our excitement from sexual imagery originates from the liver. Breath through the whole area, opening up the rib cage.

The spleen and pancreas is an earthy, golden presence that helps us to integrate. It has a singing quality.

The brain has many centers. At first, most people associate the brain with mental thought and logic. Yet, when the brain receives enough nutritive spiritual energy, the hard edge of intellectual thoughts easily dissolves into the nectars of the brain. It becomes a brilliant three-dimensional space, of which nonverbal or verbal thoughts are equally at home. The brain enters into wholeness with the rest of the body, and takes on the energy of a conduit rather than a command center. Simply put, you learn how to feel with the brain, thus removing any barriers between the brain and your heart. The brain becomes an extension of your heart and showers nectar blessings throughout the body. Start with a white color when feeding the brain.

It is not recommended that a beginner focus too much pranic energy into the heart tissues. The actual heart requires a very balanced energy, which the body knows about. Focusing too much energy in the heart can cause heart palpitations and heaviness. It is better to use the simple emotions of openness, love and compassion. General exercise is good for the heart.

An example of breathing through tissues would be around the eyes. Breathe naturally down into the lower abdomen, bring some of that breath up the spinal marrow into the head and to the third eye. Over a number of sessions gradually build up the amount of energy you can contain in the third eye area.

Feel this energy as space, liquid, soft and light. After you can build up enough presence of energy that it automatically holds your attention during the entire meditation session with no sense of headiness or headache, start to circulate the energy into the surrounding tissues. Explore all around the eyes, slowly moving the energy with your awareness through all the small muscles surrounding the eye, one at a time, try feeling inside the eyes and behind them. Feel the temples, and feel your energy having subtle nourishment, the whole session should feel refreshing and enjoyable. You may spend a half hour just exploring and vitalizing the small muscles surrounding and behind your eyes. Massage the area lightly with your fingertips from time to time.

Another example would be breathing through muscle tissue. Start by connecting with the bone nearby or underneath the muscle tissue. Feel the blood and essences within the bone potent and alive. You want to sink your energy into the bone. The bone itself is both breathable and strong. Next feel the skin above the muscles, particularly the thinness of the inner membrane of the skin. Feel that this membrane can actually be conducive to a lot of energy. Now feel the muscles themselves. They are like cotton wool, fluffy, yet tingling with vibrant electricity. They feel very open, so that any constrictions release and blood can flow through them effortlessly. Release pain in the muscle through the relaxation of openness. However perhaps unlike a general relaxation response, your attention itself does not dissipate but remains in the muscle. This attention is not static (which would create congestion) but has an alive vibrating quality to it. Visualize at times the strength of the muscle, how it can easily lift or endure. Feel the space it occupies, and breath through all this.

These examples are a start, you can make up others, but in doing so be sure to keep the energy soft and open. Visualizing pink can help with this. What you do not want is to build up too much external (raw) energy in an organ. If you do so, then you may create extra heat, or draw energy away from somewhere else that it is needed. However soft energy is unlimited, and as we gradually gain the ability to store and use it, our body can contain unlimited quantities of it. When you build up too much energy in an organ, it begins to feel uncomfortable, somewhat like if you eat too much ice cream. It may become tight, or hot. Take a nap or go for a walk. Drink some water. Singing a gentle and pleasant song will help your organs to regain their natural balance.

Each organ is surrounded by a membrane and various tissues. These tissues are meant to protect the organ.. For example the pericardium protects the heart. Much of the initial healing of our organs involves releasing built up stress from the surrounding membranes of an organ. This then enables the organ to feel more confident and contained so that it can heal form a deeper level.

Focusing into an organ can cause it to detoxify and sometimes become uncomfortable. The rule is a little at a time and gradually increase. Your body will give you all the feedback you need, provided you listen to it. Be sure to drink enough water to flush toxins (but not so much that it becomes a stress on the body to eliminate the extra water).

Always heed the warning previously given of not concentrating too much energy in the heart muscle or upper chest.

A kind of tantric mandala can be created with the energy from various organs and joints. Some advanced practitioners will actually use the subtle energy of various organs and joints to embody various enlightened spirits within their body. This overcomes illusion of the separate self and their body becomes a temple of consciousness and blessing presence. However this is not a beginning practice, for if we are not capable of creating a pure relationship with the appropriate enlightened beings then we will simply create a circus within our bodies. A pure relationship can only occur when we understand the nature of our own enlightened energy, then there is not the separation.

Spatial Awareness & Skin Breathing

Skin breathing is an excellent way to increase sensitivity that is also very healing and balancing. The skin is a third lung through which we absorb air, prana and release toxins.

Begin by sitting straight and feeling light with an easy, gentle breath. Sensitize your skin by feeling it and meditating on it. Sense the inside of your body as empty and the outside as empty. Thus your body is simply the shell of your skin. It may help to first open up and breath for a few minutes through the palms of your hands, the soles of your feet and the top of your head.

Imagine your skin to be a golden-white substance of light. This is very refreshing and balancing. In this meditation the physical breath will naturally become faint or disappear. If we desire to do skin breathing, there are several variations we can practice.

Breathing Light: Imagine nectar being poured in through the top of your head that flows over your skin. Also visualize with feeling enlightened beings surrounding you, emanating a cloud of ever-flowing prana and light. A refinement is to feel the nectar between the skin and your flesh (on the inside surface of your skin.)

Visualize this nectar light being absorbed into the tissues of your body. Use the breath to help facilitate this mixing and absorption. For example, as the light absorbs into a particular area, the breath is also used to energize that area. Thus the breath is the bridge between the light and physicality.

As you absorb the light, continually pour on more without limit. You may also visualize various colors of light-substance being painted onto your body, which is then absorbed. Be sure to give this nectar a tangible substance.

Physical Breath: As you inhale, feel yourself inhaling soft energy in through the skin, which is then absorbed by the body as you exhale. You will feel a richness and presence in the areas in which you exhale. Remember, this is not so much about inhaled air, as it is a soft energy. Thus connectivity with breath is the primary importance, and fullness of the breath is secondary.

Alternatively, exhale heaviness and toxins out through the skin. As you do this, sense a vibrant violet light all around you originating from above your head that consumes any heaviness or toxins instantly.

Subtle Breath independent of the physical breath: Absorb and release energy through the skin independently of the physical breath. One way to do this is to feel yourself simultaneously absorbing (inwards) and radiating (outwards) energy from the core of your body through the skin.

Breath of Fire

Breath of Fire, also known as bellows breathing, is rapid breathing from the navel area through the nose of about one to two times per second. Movement of the diaphragm is easy and vital with an equal inhalation and exhalation; otherwise the movement becomes forced and your navel is thrown off balance. The abdominal muscles are use to pull the navel in while exhaling and the navel area relaxes back out while inhaling. The mouth and face is relaxed (do not make a face).

Breath of Fire quickens our cellular vibration. It harmonizes the many flows of the body in one overriding rhythm and it brings the mind to an active stillness. The mind instead of following the in and out frequency of the breath, stays still. Correctly applied, this is a tremendously healing and energizing practice.

After you have become stabilized in yoga practices, have loosened the diaphragm, and mastered breath of fire for shorter times - **Try extending it first to eleven minutes,** then increase slowly to thirty-one minutes a day as a fifteen or forty day practice (woman – do not practice breath of fire on your moon cycle). As a continuous thirty-one minute practice it is recommended that you have created a feeling of wholeness through the body and have previously done consistent yogic-type practices for at least six months to one year.

Start in easy pose and incorporate various positions as necessary to move the energy and keep the breath strong. ***Maintain your mind presence*** with an awareness of free circulation throughout your body, thus continuing a strong, fluid, Breath of Fire.

Apply yourself, but do not move fanatically. If you experience strong pain, or it becomes difficult to continue the breath: Stop, relax, do some stretches to free the energy, or massage the abdomen a bit. This is not a competition. **For woman, do not do Breath of Fire on your moon cycle or if pregnant.** Also do not do breath of fire in a windy place, as it strips the energy as fast you make it.

Broken Breathing

Broken breathing is when the breath is divided into a number of distinct equal segments. This has the effect of stimulating the glandular system, increasing oxygen taken in by the body, and giving a rhythm for the mind to fall into. It also makes it easier to take a full breath when the diaphragm is not yet loosened up. The following energizing sequence is an excellent beginners technique.

Sit with a straight spine. Hands are either relaxed in your lap, one resting on top of the other or elbows against sides of the torso with fingers interlaced into a fist at the level of the heart about six to eight inches from the chest. The thumbs point straight up with their sides touching each other.

Inhale in four equal parts, Hold the breath for four counts, Exhale in four equal parts, and hold the breath out for four counts.

Mentally chant; **"Saa Taa Naa Maa,"** so that each syllable is one count, i.e., Inhale in one part while mentally sounding Saa, inhale again with Taa, etc. The four parts holding the breath is the silent sounding of Saa Taa Naa Maa.

Eyes are slightly open and looking at the tip of the nose. Do not strain the eyes, let relax and look past the nose. If it is dark, then sense the eyes looking at the nose. Inhale so the four parts completely fill the lungs; exhale so the four parts empty the lungs. **Each count is approximately one second. Start with five to eleven minutes.** After you have mastered the above, you may wish to extend to an eight part inhale, eight part hold, eight part exhale, eight part hold. You may gradually increase the time to twenty-two minutes. **Keep the mind focused on the mantra, and breathe completely and consciously.** When finished inhale and hold for about 15 to 30 seconds, exhale, stretch hands overhead, relax.

To get a feel for the mantra, practice the Sa-Ta-Na-Ma Kriya on page 104.

Pranayama for Healing & Sensitivity

Sit with a straight spine. Hold the hands in front of the chest in fists, except for the index fingers, which are straight. The right palm faces down and the left palm up as the right index finger is placed on top of the left index finger, crossing in the middle segment. Keep a light touch, so that the knuckles do not get sore.

Inhale long and deep through the nose. Exhale, slowly, through puckered lips, directing the breath at the tips of the index fingers, taking about fifteen seconds to exhale all the breath out. Feel a tingling at the fingertips. Yawning is natural as your energy is internalized. The eyes look at the crossed fingers.

Continue for ten to fifteen minutes. Then inhale deeply and hold as comfortable while continuing to look at the crossed fingers. Relax the hands after exhaling and stretch them overhead for a minute or so. Then inhale again and hold, tightening the muscles throughout the body. Isolate different muscle groups. Exhale and remain sitting for a few more minutes, feeling the benefit of the practice.

This Kriya builds a soft core of prana in the body that is very healing and uplifting. It is excellent after a day at the office, for overcoming depressive bouts, or simply as a beneficial practice. It strengthens the bone marrow and gradually recharges the body. Tensing the muscles (after finishing) draws the soft energy created from the practice further into the bones and tissues; a super health tonic!

Regular practice facilitates an intuitive sensitivity to minute changes in the "feel," or electromagnetic field both within your body and your environment, such as the weather and overall mood of your habitat.

As you gently blow the air towards your receptive fingers, also feel that you are gently blowing air through your receptive nervous system and entire body.

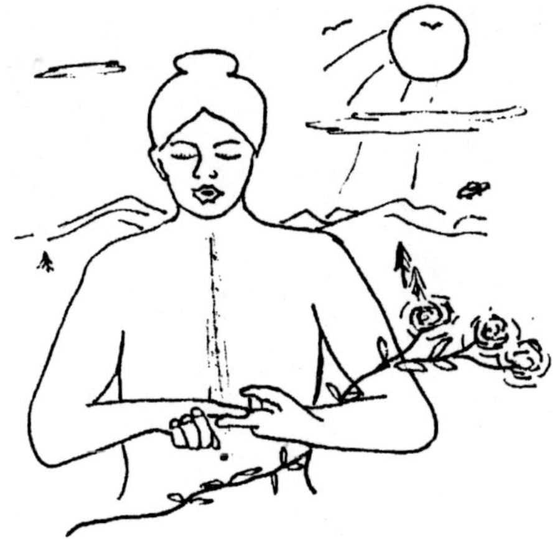

Bandu Daya Kriya

A very enjoyable and mystical kriya. When you finish everything may look smaller. This is a good practice to clear the thoughts and worries of the day. It helps to purify the blood and engage the right brain. The eight part inhale is stimulating to the glandular system in general. Practice this kriya in the evening or when you do not have any engagements afterwards.

Hold the hands in front of the chest, palms facing up. The sides of the palms touch from the base to the tip of the little fingers. Pull the thumbs back to each side. The middle (Saturn) fingertips touch, with the fingers horizontal (perpendicular to palms). All the other fingers are straight.

Inhale: **in 8 equal parts.**

Exhale: **Whistle.** Listen to the whistling sound at the third eye point (between the eyes).

Begin with eleven minutes and add one minute per day to a maximum of forty minutes.

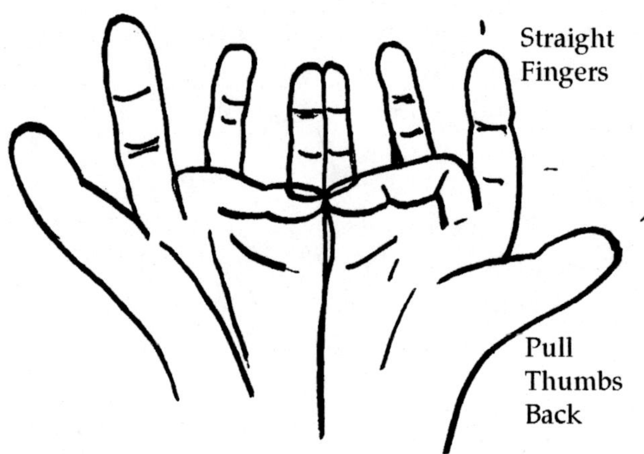

Strengthening Your Energy Body

It is advisable that a few warm-up exercises are done first. Sit with a straight spine. Extend the arms in front of you parallel to the floor with palms up. The sides of the palms are only a few inches apart. There are two ways of breathing:

Method One: Focus on the visualization, the magnetic movement of energy and breathe naturally. The arms move even more slowly than in method two, perhaps one or two minutes per cycle

Method Two: Very slowly inhale as you sweep the arms back taking 15 to 30 seconds, keeping the arms horizontal. Then **slowly** exhale as you slowly return the arms to the original position. Thus one complete breath takes from 30 to 60 seconds.

Feel the electromagnetic potency and attraction between your arms. As the arms move forward resist their attraction, which helps to build the energy. Feel prana condensing through the top of the head into the body and to the arms and hands where it mixes with energy absorbed from the hands. There is a soft ball of energy collecting at the top of the head, which has a connection to the palms of your hands. As you move your arms and hands, this moves the energy at the top of your head into a greater relationship with your body.

This should stimulate the head centers, which in turn will stimulate the navel and sexual energy. If you do not feel this, then move some of your attention downwards. The navel or solar plexus chakra must become activated before the energy can be used by the body in any quantity.

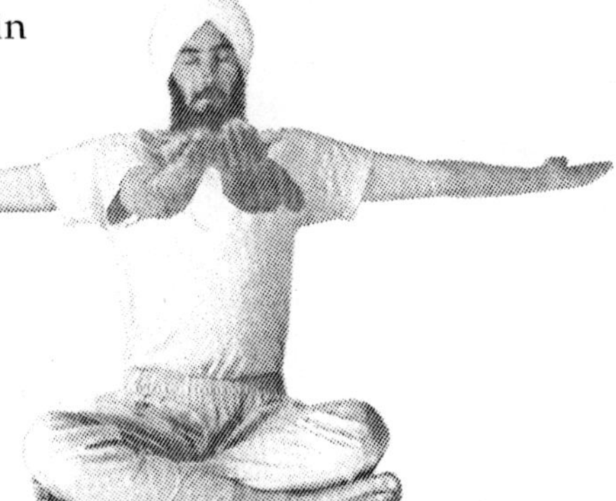

Feel a cooling, refreshing cloud of substance swirling up from the earth beneath you and into you through the increased activity of the navel area. Allow a relaxed spacious

feeling in the back of the head. The eyes are relaxed and will focus where appropriate (but do not let the mind become distracted). Every once in a while concentrate on a small bright point of light within the center of the throat. Sometimes you may want to move energy up and down through the center of the body. The building of a central core of energy in your body is a gradual and important part of the practice. Eventually the body feels as if it is swimming within itself.

As energy moves through the arms and into the spine, it will clear blockages in the shoulders and the back of the heart. This is a gradual occurrence.

Continue for 5 to 40 minutes, then relax the arms and move the hands back and forth several inches apart in front of the heart center. Look between the hands with relaxed eyes, maintaining a straight spine and neck. Build the magnetic energy between your hands. After several minutes bring the palms over the chest and breath in the energy as a blessing. Feel the balance and vitality which you have created. Then sit silently for awhile (very important).

This Kriya:

- **Recharges depleted tissues.**
- **Rebuilds and strengthens your self image.**
- **Increases the activity of the solar centers and the absorption of free energy.** This extra absorption of subtle energy strengthens the nervous system and allows the body to live on less physical food. To enhance this you may wish to visualize a golden earthy radiance and reflect that you can absorb nutritive energy from within the earth, your food, your environment, and even your thoughts.

Part of absorbing subtle energy is to coax your cells to do it. As an example, sit silently and cover yourself with liquid light, painting it on everywhere. Get into the mind-set whereby you feel this liquid light being absorbed into the physical tissues. Continue to breathe deep and full into the lower torso, while directing the soft energy of the breath into the tissues. Mix the soft energy of the breath and the painted on light together, and feel that mixing occur. You may want to focus on one area to start with. If you are absorbing the energy properly, you will feel or imagine the painted on light evaporating into the cells. Keep putting on more and more, letting it be absorbed. Give the light thickness, substance, color, tangibility. Sense the light which has evaporated into the cells, recondense into a real physical rejuvenating elixir. You can do this for as long as you want, all the while feeling more and more rejuvenated, elevated and grounded, with no sense of overload or tiredness at any time. While doing this you should also start to visualize the navel, heart, throat, and head chakras and an easy circulation between them. Feel them spatially within the body as part of the body. If you feel within your core a magnetic attraction of light, then the whole process is more effortless.

Sitali Pranayama

Sit comfortably with a straight spine and hands in Gyan Mudra (thumb and index finger touching, hands resting on the knees). The eyes are one-tenth open looking down past the tip of the nose. Curl the sides of the tongue, sticking it out through the mouth. If you cannot do this, then curl the tongue inside the mouth. Inhale, slowly drawing the breath over the tip of the tongue, feeling a cool sensation of the air drawn in over the tongue while maintaining an awareness at the spine opposite the navel. Exhale slowly through the nose (relax the mouth), maintaining an awareness at the third eye point.

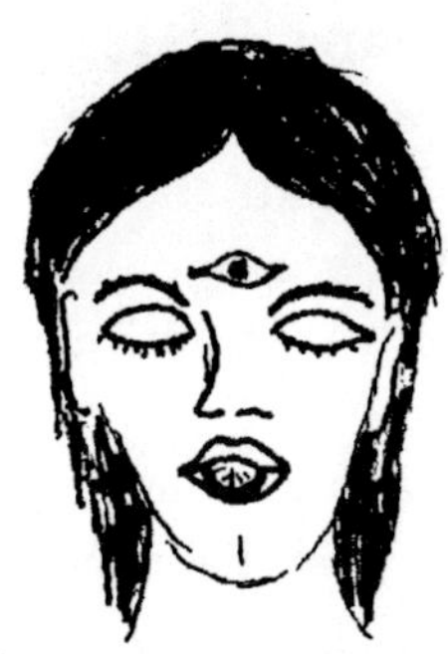

Sitali is a very cooling and tonifying practice. Excess fire energy is transmuted into the spinal marrow. Anger is transmuted into clarity and blockages are cleared, the digestive fire becomes strong, and the intuitive mind is clarified. **As a practice, repeat twenty-six times in the morning and twenty-six times in the evening.** It is said that the heavens will serve you, because your intuitive sense is opened with the sensitivity of applied breath. You will have an increased ability to create and hold a pattern of energy which organizes the ethers into a manifested reality, such as a seed creates a tree.

On Sight to Infinity

This powerful Kriya dramatically effects the physical and pranic body. It will help you to relax under difficult circumstances and move with a clarity of vision and strength. It removes the fear of death and fear in general. It stimulates and pressurizes the glands and rejuvenates the body. If you have a medically fit heart, you may use this technique to help rebuild the body to become your spiritual potential. DO NOT PRACTICE THIS KRIYA IF YOU HAVE ANY WEAKNESS OF THE HEART.

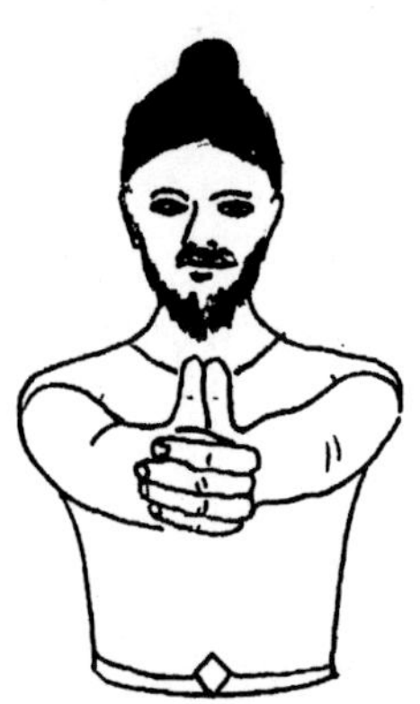

Sit with a straight spine. Extend the arms straight in front, horizontal to the ground. Wrap the fingers of the right hand over the left fist. Thumbs point straight up and are touching side by side. Look through the thumbs like a rifle sight and do not let the eyes wander.

Inhale deep taking about 5 seconds, exhale fully in about 5 seconds, hold the breath out for 20 seconds. Hold the breath out so that the body thinks it has a shortage of air. Do not leak. **Continue for 7 to 11 minutes.**

Slowly increase time to 31 minutes. After you have mastered this and practised for a month, try a few repetitions of holding the breath out for longer durations. Gradually increase duration of holding the breath out up to one minute.

Keep the back slightly rounded, so that neither the upper or the lower back is arched in. Thus the kidneys are full of energy and you do not constrict the spinal channel.

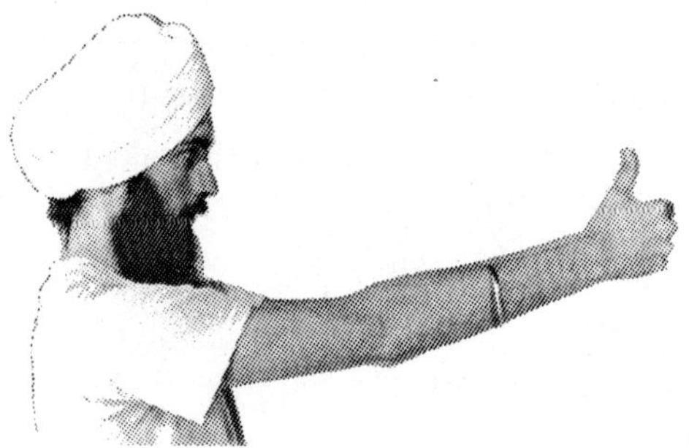

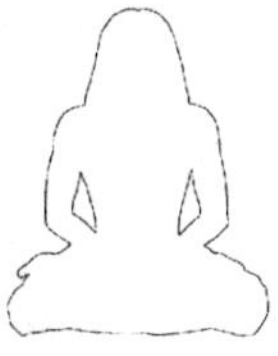

8

Chants and Visualizations

Om Ahh Hum Ha! Practice of Three Lights

This visualization is a gem that connect us with some of our chakras, essences, qualities and the enlightened presence of a master of our choosing. It is widely taught meditation within the Buddhist community. There are many refinements that can be added to it and there are many variations as to how it is taught.

In this practice we visualize a white light in the head, a red light in the throat and a blue light in the heart. At first this is simply the extent of our practice. As we get better at it, we refine the practice, so that the lights become what they actually represent (in this practice): our body, soul and spirit. An addition to the practice that I have made is at then end, drop your energy to the navel and make it more physically present, visualize a golden light for a minute and then say clearly and loudly, once, Ha! Afterwards remain silent and in the instant and non-verbal presence of total integration. This helps to crystallize the whole experience.

It should be understood that these colors are not the only colors that can be used at these centers, and that in a different context the colors can mean different things. But for the purpose of this practice, these colors and their representations are perfect.

An option, after we become adept in the basic practice is to visualize symbols within the light to maintain a focus. As an alternative to symbols, we can use miniature spheres, or if we have begun the eternal yoga practices given in the next book of this series, a miniature form of ourselves. The use of form and thus definition such as the miniature letters creates energy, which in turn supports consciousness which in full circle helps us to more effortlessly maintain our focus... Yet if our mind becomes rigid in the symbols themselves, becoming fixated on them, rather than to playfully become them, then it is better to let go and simply focus on the fluidity and beauty of radiant light.

Sit with a straight spine and simply breathe through the body for a few minutes. Feel the palms of the hands, souls of the feet and top of the head open as you bring subtle energy in through these places.

Expand bodily awareness to include the area just above the head and feel either the form of your principle guide ablaze with light or a golden-white light. Visualize this nectar-light melting into your body and rest in that for a few minutes.

In the center of your head bring forth a brilliant white light. The sphere of its origination is small, but the light itself pervades your entire body. Make it bright. Focus on the central sphere and let the pervading light emanate of its own accord. Feel the central sphere as potent, joy-filled white nectar. This nectar has substance, tangibility, and thickness. Hear the sound "Om" emanating from the nectar. As you continue, rather than looking at the light, you become it and rather than make the sound, you listen to it as yourself. You are now this light, and the body has become the environment, similar to the way we view our surroundings as our environment. In listening to the sound, do not try to hard. Initially the sound you mentally make is one of the aids to hold your attention you let go of this mental contraption and absorb yourself into a far more refined vibration that has the flavor of "Omm" or "Ahh", etc. If you are trying too hard with the sound, then shift more of the attention to the visualization of the light and relax with the sound part, or visa versa. In time it all comes together. Of all the elements, the most important is remaining within your body at the correct locations, i.e., not letting your mind wander.

Once you have established this light in the center of the head, you may choose to refocus it at the third eye point instead.

As we become this sphere of light it gains further definition, taking the form of a miniature body or a symbol representing this wonderful sound such as the letters "O". Personally I like the flowing shape of the Tibetan letter "Omm", but really it does not matter. Place a small silver-white moon-like upward facing crescent (like a little dish) above the "O" and above the crescent make a small flame. You can also use a "Om" if that connects you better to the sound. These two symbols above the letter, partly because they are small and thus very subtle, help us to connect better with our subtle body. The flame is the manifestation of our most subtle essence and the upward crescent collects the nectar form the flame simultaneously making it a tangible substance. If we choose a letter, make sure that we identify it as our body. Om represents our body and this white light is very strengthening for the body. For those who have a connection with Mahavatar BabaJi or Padmasambhava, they can visualize the white light at the third eye, about a 1/3 inch underneath the skin, with the form of Mahavatar or Padmasambhava within it. This may also be done with other personal guides.

After enjoying this for a while, let our whiteness melt and drip down into the throat, where it transforms and collects to become a brilliant deep red light that is very energetic. Again the size is small, but its brilliance pervades the entire body. This is a very mystical occurrence. This red light represents our vibrant energy nature and the throat is the center of our dream body. As we become the red light, shining in all directions, all doubt is overcome and we really begin to feel like a yogi or yogini who enjoys sitting while loosing all track of time. Everything becomes more transparent, because that is the nature of the red light. Hear the sound "Ahh" emanating from the throat filling your whole body and become this sound and its light. The sound is continual, all parts of it simultaneously present, perfection ever-expanding in the fluidity of unchanging essence. To hear this is a real let-go into our truer nature. There is passion in "Ahh," like love sounds. There is elevation is "Ahh," relaxation, beauty, enjoyment behind mental concepts. There is real energy! Tantra revolves around energy awareness. This "Ahh" is mystical because, while it ecstatically radiates, it is really dissolving everything into the center. There is a bliss of union in that implosion. It is empowered by the knowingness of the center.

After awhile, the red light drips into the heart, where it collects and forms a deep blue light. This light is very transcendental. Its sphere is very small in size; yet somehow even though it is smaller, it is bigger. There are not any boundaries to it, but at the same time you are definitely emanating out of a small area deep inside your chest, closer to your back than your front. When you think you have it, then relax, dissolve the image and telescope within to become even more transcendental, underlying everything and effortless, limitless space of radiant clear blue light. This is consciousness radiating out, which is effortless. After you have been given everything, this is all you have left. Unlike the other lights, you see it but you do not see it. It is the type of radiance that is present whether we are sleep or awake, doing something or not; it is always there. We are particularly noticing it and becoming it. The light emanates the sound of "Hum," and the sound emanates the light. The sound of hum reminds us that we are this consciousness light. This is our Spirit. Hum is the sound of we, of the universe; it contains all the answers. It is the ultimate template, one with no form, yet capable of creating any form. The more we become it, the more we feel ourselves radiating out from a little point in the middle of our heart chakra that has incredible richness around it. We are happy for no reason at all. This is real unconditional happiness. When we really begin to identify with this light, we feel incredibly empty and rich at the same time. This emptiness is the end of all our games. Become familiar with it, otherwise it can become the empty fear that stops further growth. When you embrace it, there is not a reason in the world you are not enlightened. There is nothing to do, nothing to say, and everything is done in the infinity of this radiance. A small blue letter "hum" forms spontaneously as our body. This light represents our eternal nature, our dharmakaya essence.

All three lights exist simultaneously. As we practice, we learn how to become more centered within the lights. Everything warms up within the possibility, and we sense that this is real practice; that we could even become, that we are, enlightened, liberated, and ascended, if we could just make it total. Welcome; to the everything of emptiness, the emptiness of form, the poetry of being, the simplicity of practice, the complexity of mastery, the play of tantra and the beauty of ... oh yeah, what happened to the lights, back to practice.

As a variation, imagine a master appearing and sitting in front of you, and the white, red, and blue lights emanating out of their forehead, throat, and heart and into your head, throat and heart. Feel the total intimacy of this moment, nothing is, nor can be, hidden. You and the master become one in this beautiful light.

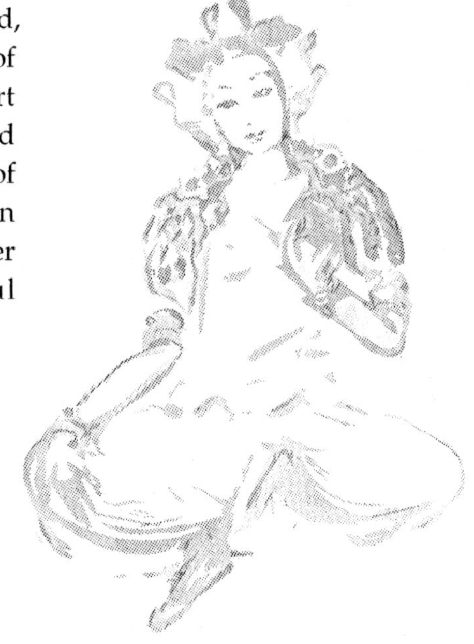

Morning Call to the Infinite

Ek Ong Kaar Sat Naam Siri Wha-He Guru

Properly done, this is one of the most powerful kundalini type kriya chants. It is definitely a high-energy experience that deepens into sacredness. It is very beautiful when several people chant together. However, if you chant it as if embarrassed, if you let your mind wander, or you do not put yourself into its entirety, then little if anything will result; most likely you will get sleepy.

It is best to do this practice on an empty stomach and after a few exercises to warm up the spine. It incorporates two and one-half breaths per one cycle of the chant. The chant moves up through the chakras; Ek at the first chakra, Ong at the second, etc. Sit straight with the hands resting on knees with the first finger and thumbs of each hand joined (Gyan mudra). Chant from 20 minutes to as long as you want (for hours). The secret is to set your self and to be mindful from the start with perfect posture; chanting clearly and not letting the mind wander for an instant. Resist any temptation to look at your watch. Keep the focus of each sound centered firmly in the body. In this way the mantra will "catch" quickly, build a considerable field of energy, and carry you into an eternal and beautiful essence of self.

When chanted in a group, the leader of the chant should keep the first syllables at a lower pitch, so as to benefit from this grounding. Just before the last round, he or she should briefly mention "last time" to indicate the final cycle of the chant. When finished, inhale deeply and hold the breath as long as comfortable. Be sure to keep you spine straight, neck locked and not to let your mind wander while holding the breath; otherwise the possible rush of energy from holding your breath will not travel through your spine correctly and you may pass out.

Inhale deeply and chant: "Ek Ong Kaar"

"Ek" Short and strong, pulling up the perineum. "Ek" means "one."

"Ong" The tongue presses up against the upper pallet as the "Ong" is sounded. Feel and imagine the sound "Ong" vibrating and emanating from the abdomen below the navel. At the same time the upper nasal and forehead is also vibrated with the sound. "Ong" is the vibratory quality of creation and also the sea of vibratory experience. All of the remaining breath is used evenly between chanting Ong and Kaar as follows.

"Kaar" Chant from the navel. Focus your attention on the sound and energy emanating from the navel chakra (like a horizontal disk). "Kaar" is the creative principle.

Chant "Ek Ong Kaar" in a lower tone. Ek Ong Kaar is attuning to the vibratory quality of creation. Every second countless thoughts pass through us from the universal thought stream or the mind of God. We ground and express those thoughts that we resonate with. "Ek Ong Kaar" is when we stop tuning in unconsciously to this thought stream, and start creating our thought as cause alone. This is another way of saying that we obtain nonverbal radiant awareness.

The oneness of "Ek" can be mystically translated as the all-pervading-ground or emptiness. In this context, "Ong" is the eternal radiance that emanates from the emptiness and Kaar is the indivisible union of radiance and emptiness, or all that we see and experience.

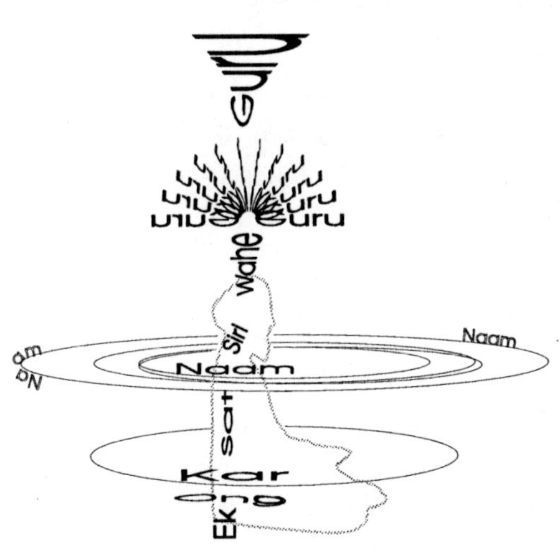

Inhale deep and chant "Sat Naam Sri"

"Sat" Short and powerful. Forcefully pull up the sound from the navel to the heart center, at the same time be aware of a calm and silent sounding in the heart for a few seconds.

"Naam" Chanted long and drawn out, using almost all the breath. This part of the mantra is one of the keys. Stay connected, feeling the sound emanate from a small radiant point in the center of the throat. Totally let yourself merge into the sound, forgetting all about the mind, thoughts, and everything else. As you continue, it will feel as if you are no longer making the sound, rather it is effortlessly and powerfully emanating from the center of the throat, dissolving yourself and all of creation into itself. It is very purifying and elevating, seducing you into the depths.

"Siri" Use the last bit of air to pop the energy up to the third eye. "Siri" is expansion, greatness and bliss, beyond what can be normally be experienced in physicality. It is a wondrous play of the intuitive consciousness applied through expression of elevating thought.

"Sat Naam" is radiance experienced as truth. It is the open door to further play and discovery, of which "Sri," blissfully and gloriously announces. The tone will probably rise in this part of the chant. As the sounding of "Naam" catches inside, it often rises considerably in pitch. While in the beginning this pitch would be uncomfortable to hold, in the later part of the chant, the high energy makes it effortless. It is important not to force this pitch, rather keep it natural, remembering to stay within the body.

"Sat" can also be mystically translated as the radiant-emptiness that is the truth of all existence. It also has the qualities of balance and penetration. It is not just the emptiness of all existence, but the ability to penetrate through the solid illusion to know this truth. Naam being identity thus describes our existence as the union of emptiness and form. Sat Naam is a sound that brings balance to the relationship of our various elemental qualities by relating form with its effortless source in the perfection.

Inhale a half breath and chant "Wha He Guru"

"Wha" Chant the sound as a rising through the top of the head, in a joyful, ecstatic way.

"He Guru" Continues above the head, like a fountain of golden white light, and rains around and through the embodiment. "He" (pronounced "Hay") means myself.

"Guru" in this understanding is not a person but the activity initiated from the eighth center above the head. Guru is awareness of our divine aspect, particularly from the budhic realms. It is the Divine stillness and the capstone of the chant. It is the stabilizing of your expanded understanding as a deeper and more fulfilling reality of life. As the word "Guru" is sounded feel a timeless still feeling of hearing all parts of the word at the same time, everywhere. The pitch usually lowers on the sounding of Guru, and a remembrance of the sound continues, as the energy rains down the body and you inhale fully to start the mantra the next cycle of the mantra. Do not let the mind wander as Guru rains down through and around the body, while you inhale to start again; otherwise the chant will not build in its power.

For the energy to properly build there are two important key points. The first is in the sounding of Naam. As the energy builds in the various chakras and pathways, it is the opening of the throat that will shift the energy to become self-sustaining and seductively encompassing. The sounding of Naam is a total surrender into ecstatic emptiness, a total let-go. The second key point is in the sounding of Guru, through subtlety, purity and totality. It is here, that the Kriya moves beyond entertainment and into the blissful eternity of self.

This meditation is a total surrender into the "will of the One" through vibrational alignment, purity of the chant, and stimulation of the Kundalini. It is a complete and wonderful formula. **Chant it strongly and consciously, so as to physically and subtly vibrate inside the body.** Give meaning to the chant through the power of your soul. This chant when done sacredly opens the chakras for a genuine experience. Enjoy!

Sa-Ta-Na-Ma Kriya of Sounds

This wonderful Kriya washes the mind, adjusts the elemental balance in the body, gradually develops a relationship with your presence above the head and increases projection, presence and healing ability.

For all these benefits, it is a simple practice, but must be done daily for the accumulative effect. Practice for a minimum of forty days. Some days it is heaven, others, not much at all seems to happen. Take heart that during the not-much-happening-days, if you can keep the sincerity of focus at this time it is perhaps doing the greatest good, literally penetrating through subtle resistance and rewiring the brain.

Sit with a straight spine, in a meditative composure. Eyes are marginally open looking downward, keeping the tip of the nose in view. Do not strain the eyes, as it is a subtle connection. This downward glance helps your centering in the body, at the same time stimulating the region between the eyes and keeping you internal.

Feel, activate, or simply imagine a continual beam of light-presence from above your head entering the body. For this particular Kriya, direct most of the light to the center of the head (pineal gland) and then turn it ninety degrees and let it project out through the forehead, into infinity. Keep this visualization going throughout the practice.

Rest your hands on knees and begin chanting:

As you chant:

Saa Press thumb and first finger together.
Taa Press thumb and second finger together.
Naa Press thumb and third finger together.
Maa Press thumb and little finger together.

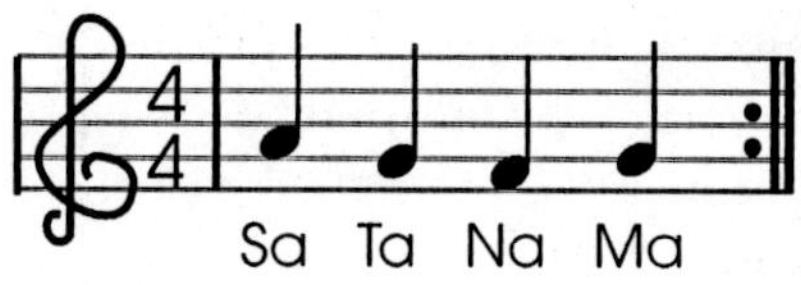

All the sounds are pronounced as in "ma." Keep going in this cycle, letting the breath adjust itself automatically. Every once in a while, sense that the energy required to touch the thumbs and fingers together originates from the navel region. Create a disk of light around the waist and sense it traveling up through the body, out the arms and to the fingers.

Chant in the following format of three voices:

5 Minutes	Normal voice
5 Minutes	Whisper
11 Minutes	Silent (continuing inwardly)
5 Minutes	Whisper
5 Minutes	Vocal
31 Minutes Total	

During the silent part, keep the mantra inwardly going, along with the visualization and movement of the fingers. Switching through the different voices helps the penetration of your wakeful state into the subtle realms and back again with full recollection and integration. The whispering has a sense of etheric penetration, a voice of longing, of lovers. During the silence keep the mind on the mantra, going deeper into your soul.

When finished, inhale deeply and hold the breath, channeling presence up the spine. Be particularly sure to keep the neck straight, chin slightly tucked in and the mind focused. Hold as long as comfortable. As you release the breath be sure to keep the neck lock, as there can be a real rush of energy. If so, tighten muscles around the spine and neck to contain the energy so you do not get dizzy. Sit quietly for a few minutes, then stretch the hands overhead for a few seconds.

Additional Refinements

Feel the mantra originating on a current of light from above the head. As you say each syllable, it descends into the head and exits through the forehead into infinity. Do not follow the sound; rather let it go.

If you are able to hear the internal tones, then try feeling the current of light also as this current of sound. As you say each syllable, let its sound originate from the sound current, again a few inches to a foot above the head, then down and out through the forehead. When this happens you will be listening to the chant as much as you are saying it.

Meaning of the Mantra

It is advisable to simply focus on the sounds in their vibratory quality. Do not let the mind move around too much in intellectual meaning. This helps you to simply be present in a deep way with the practice. As you are able to hold this, then you can bring in an additional richness through understanding the meaning of each syllable, letting the mantra become the embodiment of that quality.

Saa is the infinite sea of our light presence, radiant emptiness.

Taa is bringing forth an image, a definition, or a point of focus within that light. It also means "yes," and is a reference to the Goddess and the light at the third eye.

Naa is purification, alignment and elevating our vibratory consciousness to accept and integrate this light being brought forth into our life.

Maa is the birth, the manifestation of this light into our world.

Together ***Sat*** is our god-head, the eternal radiant presence, or simply truth. ***Naam*** translates as our identity. Together Sat Naam means *"I Know my Eternal Self-Radiant Identity,"* or *"I AM Radiant,"* or *"Emptiness and Form,"* traditionally simplified as "I AM Truth."

This meditation tells the story of the eternally radiating light of the sea of emptiness being consciously qualified into identity, the preparation for that light to be integrated into existing creation and finally the joy of manifest creation. In Buddhist terms, Saa is the universal grounds of the dharmakaya. Taa is for lack of a better word, our soul within the dharmakaya coming into sambhogakaya. Naa is our sambhogakaya image coming into nirmanakaya (physicality). Maa is the bliss of the continuum, the mother of creation in oneness (emptiness).

Hunsa (Swan) Kriya

This Kriya is said to bring the expanse and experience of many lifetimes. It stimulates the pineal and pituitary glands and opens the third eye through regular practice. It is best practised at night, preferably sitting in bed just before lying down.

Curl the fingertips into the palms (touching the finger mounds). Palms facing forward, bring the hands approximately six inches in front of the eyes. The thumbs press together and are pointing down, joined in their last cubit. Look at the thumbtips and fix their image in your sight. Then close the eyes and continue to see the thumbtips through the closed eyes as pure white light. Open your eyes if necessary to regain the image. After a few minutes the arms will feel locked in place, which helps you to transfer awareness more to your electromagnetic field. You may feel as if the thumbtips are coming in through the top of the head.

Start with five to seven minutes and slowly increase the time through your internal sense of when to stop.

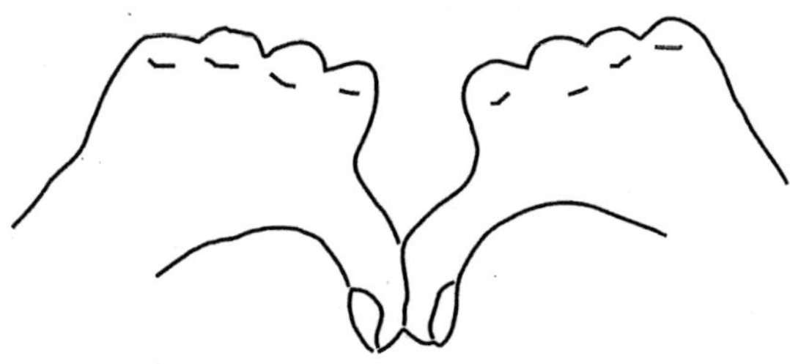

Ecstatic Presence of Life Kriya

Be sure to sit with a straight spine. This Kriya increases internal voltage, purifies and heals the body, and makes us feel very alive. In this state, it is easy to mix the aliveness of ourselves with an increased flow of energy to awaken the central channel flowing up through the body. You can discover for yourself secrets hidden within the body such as nectars" kissing" at your navel chakra, the cave of unparalleled beauty and vibrational resonance within the center of the brain, the inner rain, and indescribable presence of awakened awareness...

Sit in a meditative posture. Bring the hands into a bear grip in front of the thymus gland with the left palm facing in. Twist the left hand, so that both thumbs are pointing down, and press the thumb tips together. The twist of the hands provides a stimulation which helps to keep you awake and alert enabling you to better channel prana into the spinal column and activate the upward movement of energy. Concentrate at the brow point between the eyes. However, never let the energy feel top or bottom heavy. This is done by keeping both the head and navel areas open and thus a circulation between them. It is also done by deepening and softening the buildup of energy so that it has an inner dimension in which to expand.

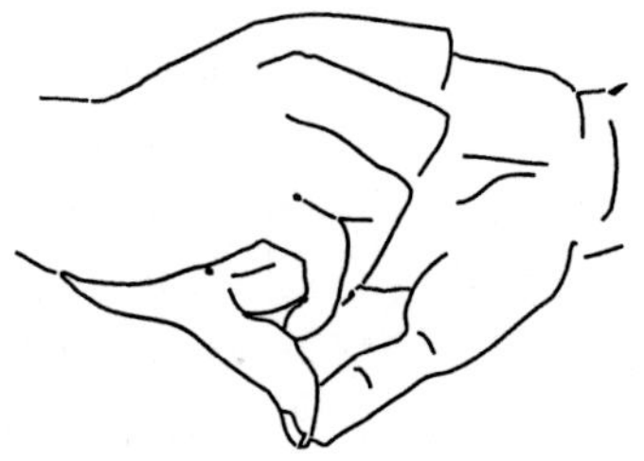

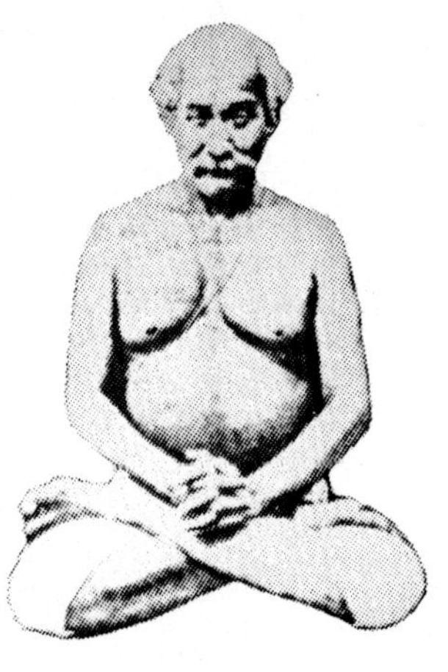

By energetically chanting with totality; inner alertness, abundance of prana and meditative direction are all harmonized as a quickening within every cell. Thus the spiritual dimension of your body can be realized.

Take a deep breath and chant (in one breath):

" Ra Ra Ra Ra
Ma Ma Ma Ma
Rama Rama Rama Rama
Sa Ta Na Ma"

Chant at a pace where it takes all the breath to do the chant, usually about 20 to 40 seconds. Practice daily for 22 minutes.

For those who are experienced in a steady practice and understand the transformative and sometimes challenging effects that longer pranayama can create in the body and emotions, you may gradually build the time to 2-½ hours for the full effect. When finished, inhale deeply and hold the breath as long as comfortable at the navel. For the full time, part of the Kriya may be done in silence.

Raj Mudra
a nice bedtime practice

Sit with a very straight spine. Place the hands in front of the heart. Cup the hands so that the sides of the middle, ring, and little fingers touch. The little fingers are closer than the other fingers. Finally touch the index finger and thumb together as in Gyan Mudra. Arms are relaxed by the sides. Eyes are part way open, looking at the tip of the nose and seeing the hands as well.

Hold the posture in silence, allowing the breath to adjust naturally. Meditate silently for about fifteen minutes before going to sleep.

"Raja" means king or royal and this mudra facilitates a centering within oneself and the beautiful regality of that.

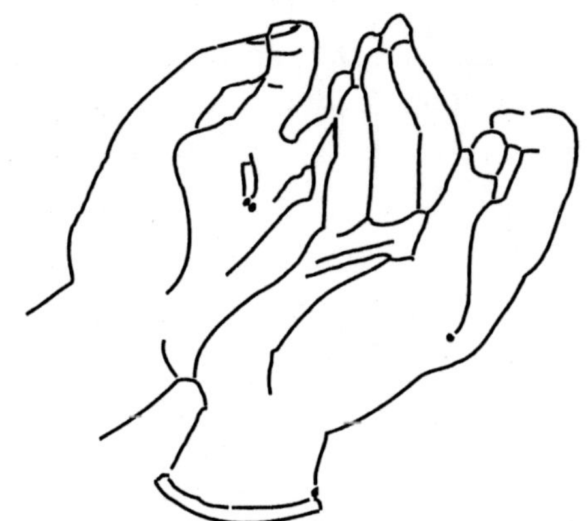

Piercing the Inner Veils

This Kriya purifies misunderstanding and awakens a continual and profound sense of inner radiance originating from within. It brings an experience of purity. Intellectuality is overcome and you are able to both speak from the heart and hear what is really being said underneath all that is spoken to you. By continuing to cultivate the inner space this practice opens you enter the rarefied realms within the heart. As the heart becomes pure, everything is seen as connected to the "one" or highest self of all, despite contradictions which may appear in outer life. It is a very blissful practice.

This is a good practice to do as a preliminary to subtle tantric meditations within the heart and the surrounding channels, such as taught in the completion stages of tantric meditation.

Bring the hands in front of the Heart center and interlock the thumbs. The left palm faces flat down, the right palm faces forward. The two hands are at a 90 degree angle to each other.

Inhale and powerfully chant :

"ONNGGG KAARA"

Focus either in the heart or the throat center. Sense a small sphere of clear-like light originating from that point, and reside within that point. The "ONG" is very forceful — like a vibrating machine. Feel the vibration in the guts, the head, and most important, feel the purity of the sound in the heart center. Finish with a short "Kaara." "Kar" rhythms with "car" except the "r" is more of a hard sound as the tongue flicks against the upper pallet. As the tongue leaves the upper pallet a short and slight "a" sound follows, with a sense of going forward in time and space.

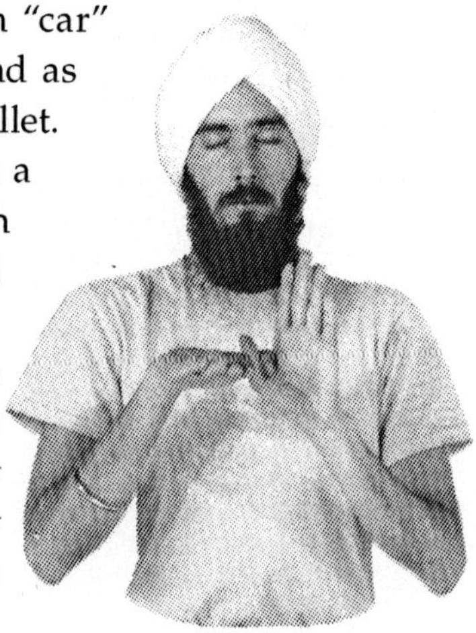

Start with 11 minutes, practice for a week or two, then increase to 45 minutes for a minimum of six weeks. In every repetition use all your attention to really vibrate the "ONG" sound and put some power behind it. It may take a few weeks for the throat to adjust and thus it is wise to build the time gradually. If you vibrate the mantra as such it will definitely cause the glands to secrete, giving a feeling and chemistry of youth, freshness and purity. Intensity also keeps the mind focussed. Be sure to internalize the sound at the same time that you are giving external force to it.

When finished chanting, inhale deep, hold the breath, apply the locks, and slightly tighten the back of the neck. Hold as long as comfortable. Exhale and relax the breath. Remain very still and in the after effect. Then stretch the hands over head and move the body a bit, feeling the simplicity and happiness of life. Become the conscious creator of thought, as well as the receiver of thought. "Ong" is the infinite sea of vibration as it manifest into form. "Kaar" is the creation that comes forth from this infinite sea. Thus Ong Kaar is radiant form and formless radiance, the one taste, also known as Ati.

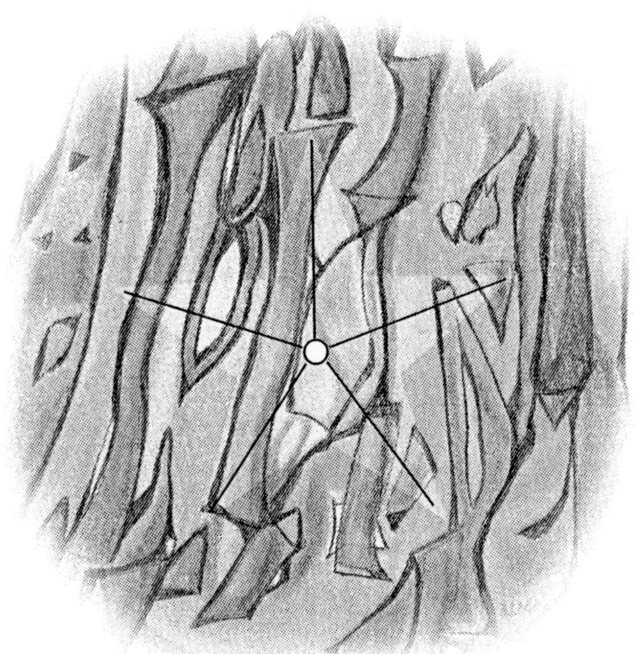

Throat Chakra Kriya

ONG KARA ONG KARA ONG KARA ONG

PART ONE: Sit with a straight spine. Hold the hands about six to eight inches in front of the throat and interlace the ring and middle finger so they point in toward the body (palms facing in). The little finger and index finger fold flat over each other. The thumbs point straight up. Press the pads of the two fingers pointing in, against each other with a strong pressure. The forearms are parallel with the floor and the elbows are out to the sides. The eyes are slightly open looking at the tip of the nose. Chant the following for 11 minutes at a fairly rapid pace (about eight seconds per round including a short inhale in the beginning).

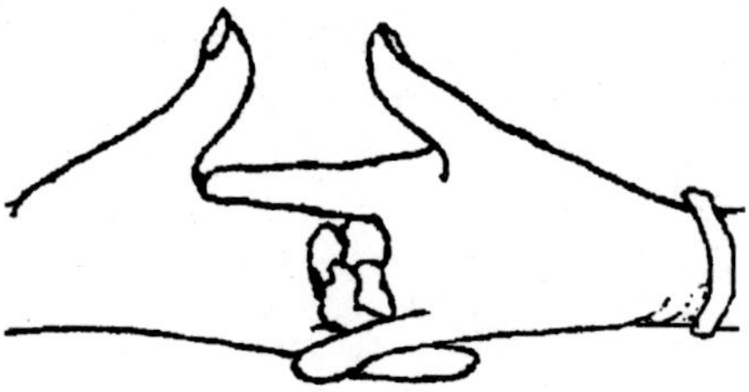

"ONG KAR ONG KAR ONG KAR ONG"

The "ONG" has the emphasis. "KAR" rhythms with "car," except the "R" is a hard "r," so that a slight "a" sound will result in the end ("KARa") as the tongue leaves the upper pallet and prepares to sound the next syllable.

This Kriya is very effective if you put yourself into it. Make sure to keep the middle fingers firmly pressed together. When finished, inhale and hold the breath at the navel as long as comfortable, keeping the hand position. Relax the hands after exhaling.

PART TWO: Forget about the breath and bring all your attention within the center of your throat as a small sphere about 1/4 inch in size. Make it red or blue in color, and concentrate in being inside and as the sphere radiating out (not from the outside looking in). To achieve this you have to be alive as the sphere, rather than a mechanical activity.

Stay with this for some time. This Kriya is particularly good in the evening before going to sleep. It will make the pressures of the world seem less. It helps awaken the throat center, which when related to the rest of the body, brings subtle nourishment and increases bliss.

Mental Clarity

This practice cleanses and strengthens the organs, increases internal pressure, clears and sharpens the mind, and through continued practice; everything around you sounds like a song.

Sit with a straight spine. Make the left hand into a loose fist at heart level about eight inches out from the body. Wrap the fingers of the right hand in a fist over the left. The fingers of the right hand do not go past the knuckles of the left. Fold the right thumb over the left. Moderately tighten the fists and keep the pressure.

Eyes may be either slightly open looking at the tip of the nose, the third eye point, or closed looking through the top of the head. Be sure to keep a good grounding at your navel chakra.

Chant five times on a single breath :

"Wahe Guru Wahe Guru Wahe Guru Wahe Jio"

for 11 to 31 minutes. To experience the mystical benefit, chant 31 minutes a day for three months.

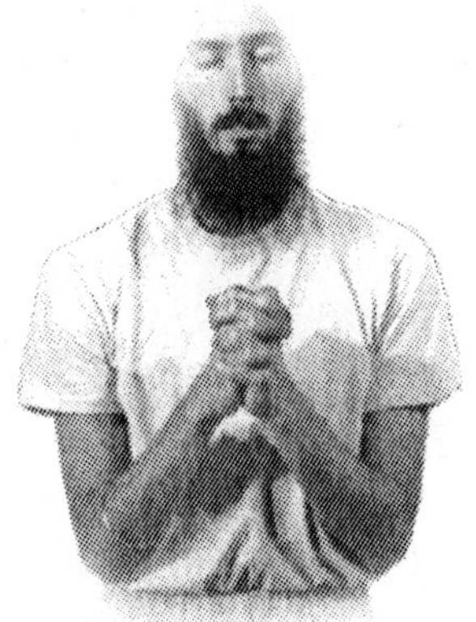

Note: This picture show the hands folded in a different way. Follow the instructions as given in the text above.

Meditation for Transformation

This Kriya can clear deep obstructions, somewhat like the sun burning through clouds. It requires a yogic attitude of perseverance, but if that is you, then it is a wonderful practice that can develop a vibratory power. Keep in mind that techniques can clear obstructions, but must be blended with the ever flowing life experience of love before they have any potency of bringing forth your soulful beauty. This Kriya can help you break through struggle into an experience of effortlessness.

Sit straight and bring your hands to the level of the solar plexus. Extend the index fingers forward and touch the tips together. Extend the thumbs up and back. The base of the hands and thumbs touch the body. Keeping the neck straight, open the eyes a bit and look down at the hands. Inhale deep and chant up to 40 times on a single breath.

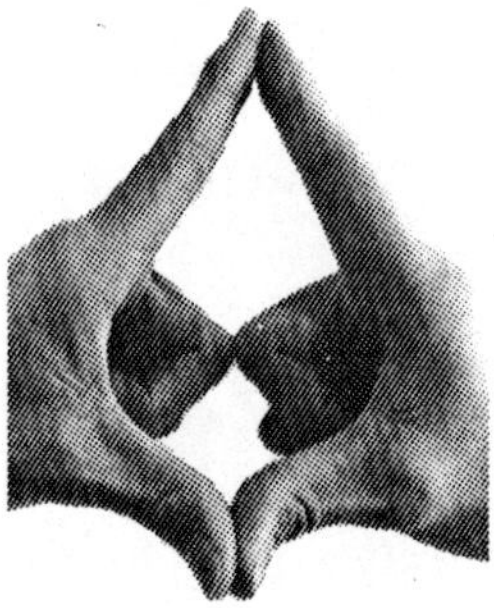

"Wahe Guru"

Chant so the sounds are distinct and in a three part rhythm of "Waa-Hay-Guroo." Try it for a few minutes with an exaggerated pronunciation so as to understand the movement of the tongue and mouth. You may need to start with 16, 20, 24, 28 ... Repetitions and gradually increase with your capacity. Use the last bit of air in each breath cycle and do not take in extra air to finish.

Start with 11 minutes and slowly increase to one half or one hour. Do not put undue pressure on your body by forcing yourself beyond the number of reps per breath you can do or a longer overall time than your body can integrate. This is not only uncomfortable, but diminishes the deeper benefits of the Kriya, because the strain interferes with a natural channeling of energy into the inner channels. Woman on their moon cycle (or if pregnant) should not do this type of kriya.

Practicc for three to six months to gain greater benefit.

Rhythm for the Night

This kriya is a good practice before bed. Its rhythm stays with you and cleanses the mind while sleeping. Sit with a straight spine and hands in Gyan Mudra.

Inhale fully in four equal parts mentally chanting:

"Sa Ta Na Ma" (a syllable on each inhale)

Hold the breath for four cycles of mentally chanting:

"Sa Ta Na Ma" (total of sixteen counts)

Exhale fully in two equal parts while mentally chanting:

"Wahe Guru"

For a total of twenty-two equal counts.

Start at 7 to 11 minutes and **gradually** increase to 31 minutes. Do not practice if you are too tired or exhausted. If you feel a little tired, start the practice and if you do not feel fully awake after five to ten minutes, stop and sit silently until you go to sleep.

Keep the tongue pressed against the upper palate behind the teeth. Project the mantra through the third eye point. Press fingers firmly in Gyan Mudra. Press the breath down into the lower abdomen. If you start to get slightly dizzy while holding the breath; make sure the tongue is pressed up, apply Mhula Bhand and squeeze the buttocks and muscles around the spine including the neck. If you get noticeably dizzy, stop, and do something else, such as a few stretches, drink some water, relax.

Dizziness comes when energy is not held within the energy channels of the body. Thus squeezing muscles helps to direct energy back into the body. Also it takes awhile for the body to adjust and this should never be rushed.

Options:

- If holding for 16 counts is too difficult, then hold for eight counts instead.
- After exhaling in two parts while mentally chanting Wahe Guru, you can either immediately inhale in 4 parts to begin the next cycle, or else hold the breath out for an additional 2 counts before beginning again (with silence).

Ah-Uu-Om Kriya of One

This very sacred and wonderful Kriya brings understanding and harmony of vibratory expression within many levels of your being. It realigns the body to its etheric counterpart and brings a skeletal alignment in the upper spine and shoulders. A golden quality develops around a person practising this Kriya and there comes the sharpness and ability to integrate many aspects of life into a feeling of a synchronistic whole.

This brings an ability to confidently communicate at various frequencies of vibratory existence. New experiences are more easily assimilated and indeed the integration includes the guts, heart, and head. Through continued practice various etheric centers opening up in a dynamic relation to each other in a soft silk like ecstatic radiance. Perhaps what is most remembered is the coziness and simplicity from surrender into oneself that this Kriya facilitates.

There is no need to bring forth an analytical translation, of the mantra, because it is of the sound current. Light and sound integrate as an emotionally felt pulsation of bliss. For those who are surrendered into the transmission of practice, there is timeless rest in every syllable and ecstasy in the coming of the next syllable.

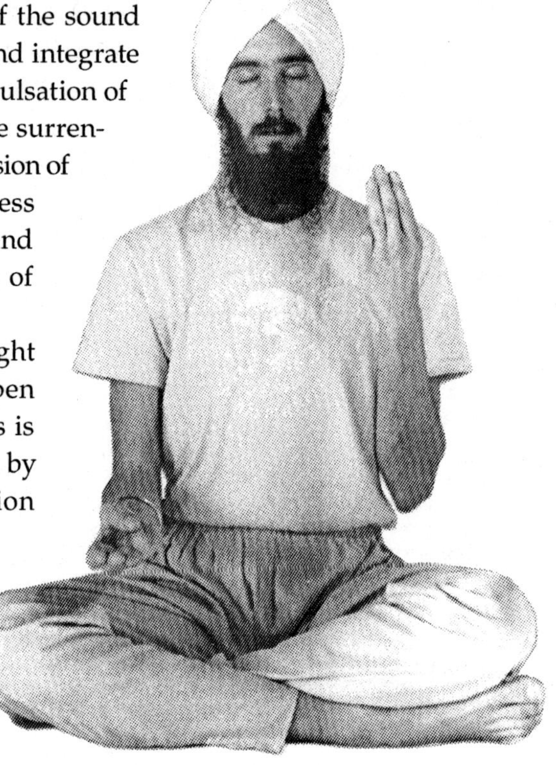

Sit with a straight spine. Eyes may be open or closed, but the focus is within. Elbows relaxed by the sides, just a fraction of an inch forward, giving a sensation of forwardness. Forearms straight out in front, palms flat and facing up.

Hold the tip of the little finger with the thumb (Bhuddi Mudra). The remaining fingers are straight.

Chant "Ah" : as the left hand moves up.

Chant "Uoo" : as the right hand moves up and the left hand moves down.

Chant "oM" : as the left hand moves up and the right hand moves down.

Silence : as the left hand moves down and the right hand moves up.

Continue, in a fluid rhythm (not jerky). Pace may be rapid or moderately slow, but keep it fairly consistent. A rhythm about that of a calm heartbeat is recommended. The wrists do not bend. From the elbows to the shoulders (and the body) remains stationary. Say the sounds very distinctly and totally dissolve your mind into their sounding and thus presence. If any part of the mind starts going off in a tangent, then have that part chant the mantra. **Make the sounds in the back of the throat.**

Time : 15 to 45 minutes.

Being in that which always is

Tratakum

The practice of visual focus upon a image or point is called "Tratakum." It is an aspect of kriya and meditation practice which:

- Strengthens the eyes.
- Brings out and increases internal energy.
- Helps to balance the two sides of the body and the brain hemispheres.

While fixing your focus upon an object keep the eyes soft, yet penetrating and unmovable. Retain an upward energy moving out through the eyes as if looking at someone you love very much. Do not become mesmerized into an unconscious trance, zombie like. You may experiment with connecting energy from your heart, liver, kidneys or another organ to your eyes.

While engaging in tratakum keep the posture regal and the spine straight. As the breath automatically deepens, occasionally apply Mhul Bhand a bit to increase the internal circulation of energy, that arises from the intensity of focus.

Tratakum gives a focus and locks the wandering of our visual sense. As the eyes fix in place, they do not look this way or that, which arouses attention of the mind. This brings a natural state of meditation which brings you first through purification and aligning, and then deeper experiences of the self.

The practice of tratakum may reveal the divinity present within all, as all is present within. Following are a few beginning practices. When you are finished, blink your eyes rapidly for a minute and perhaps gently massage around the eyes.

More advanced tratakum practices include the ability to physically influence what you are looking at, such as moving a candle flame.

Meditating Upon a Leaf or Object in Nature

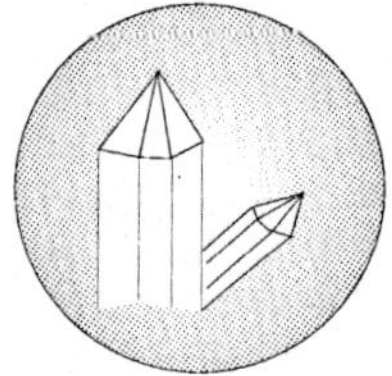

Sit in an area of nature, preferably in the shade where the light is not too strong and find a leaf or small object in front of you and fix your focus on it, not wavering an inch for about ten to fifteen minutes. Let the eyes water if they do so, it is very cleansing. The breath will automatically deepen.

Looking at a Candle Flame

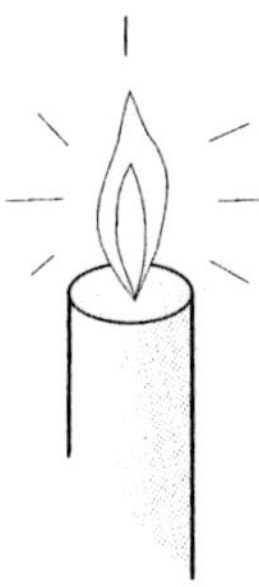

Set a candle on a table and fix your focus on it for ten to fifteen minutes. Try fixing your focus on different parts of the flame. At some point you may feel that the image of the flame exist inside your head and yet you still see it where it is. Remain alert to the movement of the candle.

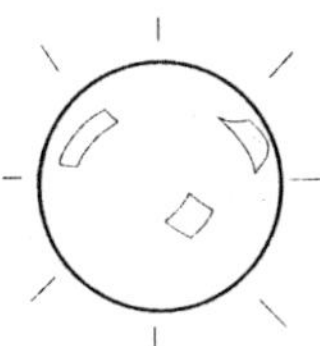

Healing From the Sun

Take in the healing energy of the sun for a few minutes during sunrise and sunset. Do not look at the sun when more than two diameters above the horizon.

Massaging the Eye Muscles with Energy

Close the eyes, or open them 1/10th, while remaining relaxed. Learn to bring a focus of energy at the third eye and within that energy make it soft and nectar like. Pink helps with this. For some people this first step might take many short sessions, because tension needs to be released so that this energy can remain soft and you do not experience a headache.

Breathe normally and consciously so that you guide some of the energy of your breath to increase nectar energy at the third eye. Then slowly start to spread it out. Start with the base and sides of the nose, extend it across the forehead to the temples. As you spread the energy feel it move both on the skin, under the skin, through the muscles and inside the bones of the face. Pay attention to small details and a three dimensional sense. Feel the energy gently pushing outwards, i.e., it is radiant, so as to open up a space of lightness. Always keep the center at the third eye; if you loose it come back to it, center, and then spread out again.

Next move the energy through the eyelids, taking your time, then under the eyes, through the cheeks, behind the eyes, through the jaws, etc. As you slowly move your attention, feel a slight tingling of energy and its movements. Remember to gently extract energy from the breath by breathing down into the lower abdomen. Repeat movements of energy through the various small muscles around the eyes, in the eyes, and behind them. This is a very refreshing and enjoyable exercise that makes you feel younger.

Body,

Mind,

and Breath

is the golden formula brought

together in the skilful science

of Kriya Yoga

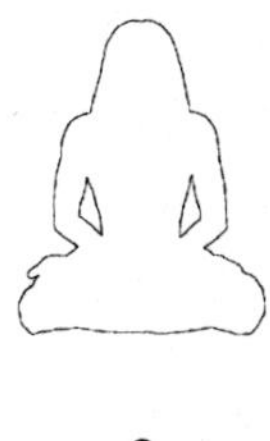

9

Dynamic Yoga Sets

Dynamic Yoga Sets are a great way to increase energy, remove agitation, clear blockages and prepare us for deep meditation. This type of yoga is also an excellent form of active meditation.

These sets can be done either in silence or to music. If you are not limber enough for a particular exercise, then modify it or do the best you can. Times given are general; again modify them so that they work for you. When first starting out, be sure to leave enough time when you are finished to relax on our back. More experienced practitioners may choose to go directly into a sitting mediation or a kriya.

Remember to maintain presence with what you are doing. If your mind wanders, come back and remind yourself to stay present. Maintaining awareness of the breath in relation to the body helps ours focus. Adding a mantra on the breath, such as "Sat" while inhaling and "Naam" while exhaling can make everything into a magical flow of the present.

In this yoga we breathe deeply and at times a little exaggerated. The extra energy is assimilated through the exercises and our grounding into cellular vibrancy. However, if you get dizzy, please slow down or stop until you are no longer dizzy. No benefits obtained by continuing in a dizzy state.

When this type of yoga is done as a discipline, it has the capacity to bring up our resistance and emotional stuff. For those who have or want the blessing of intensity, the best approach is to keep moving, go through it, and remember your depth. This does not necessarily mean that you have to overdue it, just keep moving in a graceful, empowered and alert way. Experience the purity of radiance, the joy of being. As an analogy, if you felt exhausted, grimy, hungry, disorientated; is this the best viewpoint to see clearly. When our body and minds are full of toxins, it is similarly difficult to get a clear perspective. First get the clarity, then from that place see what you need to see, and change what you need to change. The rest just takes care of itself.

Be sure to read the earlier chapters, particularly guidelines for practice, and locking and containing energy in the body.

Brightening Your Aura

Your radiance and the invisible field of effect you carry and project must be able to gracefully prepare your way. When you feel light and bright, your energy is then a source of inspiration and healing. If your presence does not work, then life becomes a struggle. Release the struggle, with the ease that results when you have enough energy and inspiration, by brightening your radiance with this set.

Vital to the whole process is deep strong breathing; to clean the blood, clear blockages, and increase your voltage. You bring the final refinement through the qualifying power of your goodness.

The Long Warm Up is a great set in itself. For **a shorter warm-up** do exercise #1, 4, 5, 11 and 12.

LONG WARM UP

1) Circle, Up and Around: 1 minute

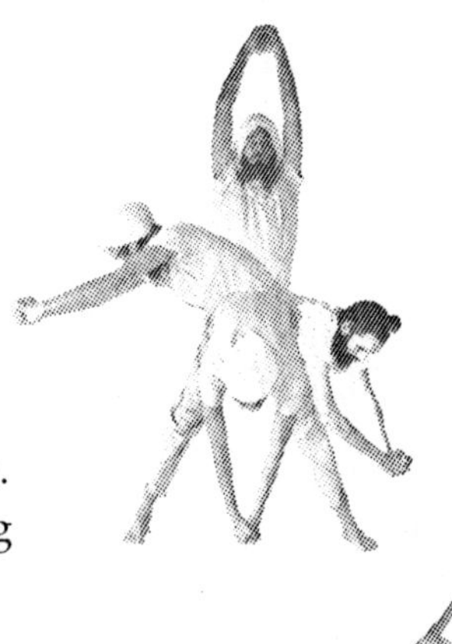

Stand up with the legs several feet apart. Interlace hands together into a fist. Bend down, inhale as you sweep the arms up and over the head and exhale as they continue their sweep full circle to the original position. Then reverse direction and continue. Big smooth arcs.

2) Standing backward stretch: 1 to 3 minutes.

Remain standing, stretch the arms overhead. Hold the little finger down against the palm with the thumb. Lean back with the whole body. Eyes open. Feel a stretch across the upper chest and thymus.

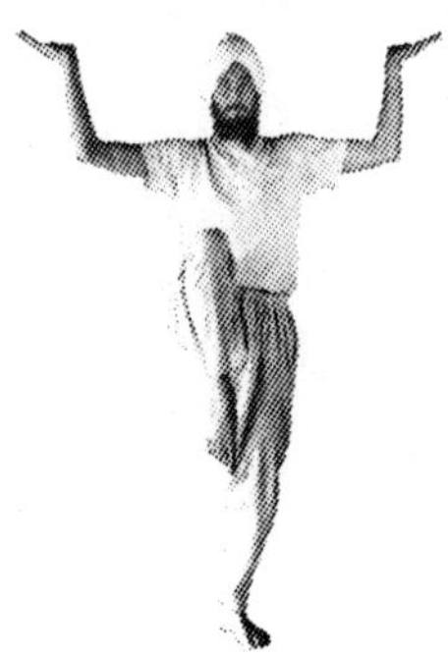

3) Yogi Walk : 1 to 5 minutes

Standing with both arms out to the sides, bend the arms so that the forearms are straight up, then bend the wrist 90 degrees so palms are facing the sky. Inhale alternate knees to the chest.

4) Dynamic Life Nerve Stretch: 2 to 3 minutes

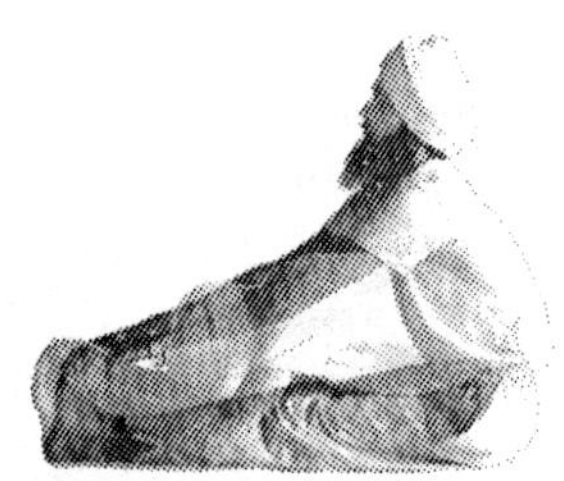

With legs extended in front, grab the toes, or however far you can reach while keeping the legs straight. Inhale up, exhale as you stretch down. As you inhale up, the head will naturally tilt back a bit. Dissolve the activity of the mind into the motion and breath as you mentally chant "Sat" on the inhale and "Naam" on the exhale. When finished, exhale down, inhale deep and hold the breath for 15 to 30 seconds, not moving a single muscle.

5) Leg lifts: 1 to 3 minutes, then hold legs straight up for 1 minute

Lie on the back. Inhale both legs up, exhale down. Keep the lower back pressed against the floor.

This helps to strengthen the navel area and transmute energy up the spine. A connected navel energy makes it much easier to hold a focused intention. During the day at spontaneous times and before going to sleep feel the area of the spine opposite the navel as open and sparkling.

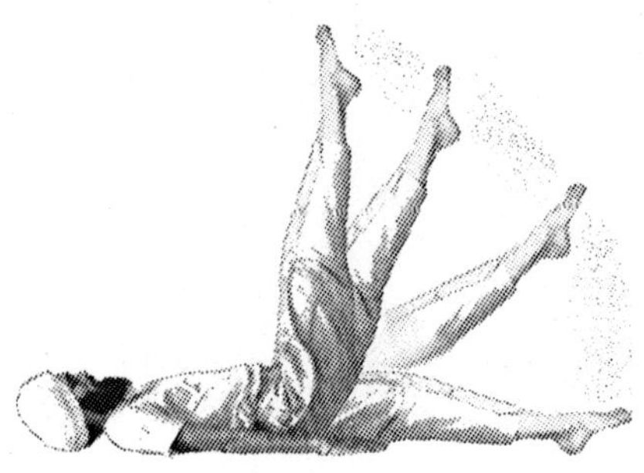

6) Nabhi Butterfly : 3 minutes

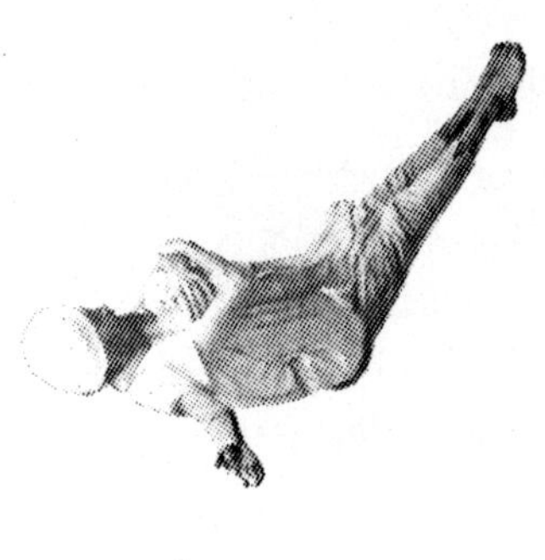

Remaining on the back, bring the knees to the chest and wrap the arms around the knees, holding them to the chest. Inhale as you unfold the arms to the ground and straighten the legs to a 45 degree angle. Exhale to original position. Feel the exercise with a meditative connectivity to the movement and breath.

7) Relax on back : 2 to 5 minutes

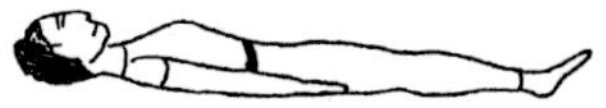

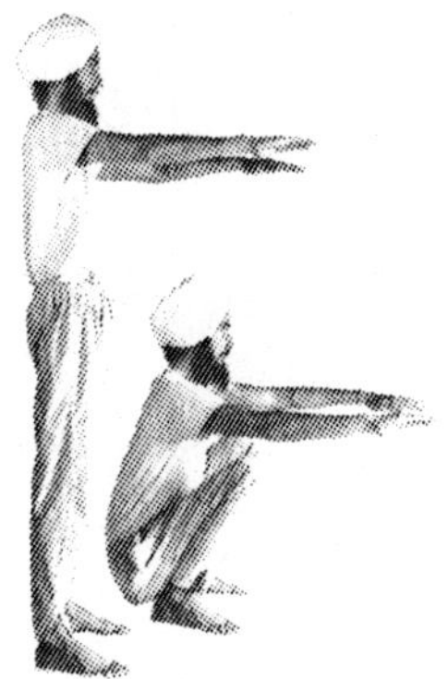

8) Squats with arms in front : 10 to 26 repetitions

Squat with arms held straight out in front, shoulders relaxed. Inhale up, exhale down.

9) Blessing the Earth : 1 to 5 minutes

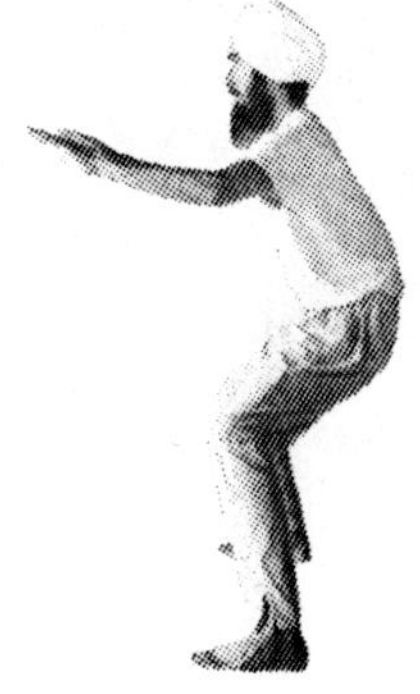

Stand with the feet about three feet apart. Arms straight in front and 45 degrees to the sides with palms facing down. Bend the knees into a stance. Keeping the knees bent, move the torso from side to side as you gently bounce up and down. Sink down, as you face left, center, and right, bouncing up in-between. Feel yourself blessing the earth as you participate in a sacred dance.

10) Chant "Ma" for 11 minutes

Sit with a straight spine. Look at and past the tip of the nose, eyes only a little open. Place both hands flat, palms up, on top of each other and against the body at the solar plexus. Thumbs point straight outward from the body. Men place the right hand on top of left and women place the left hand on top.

Continuously chant in a monotone "Ma"

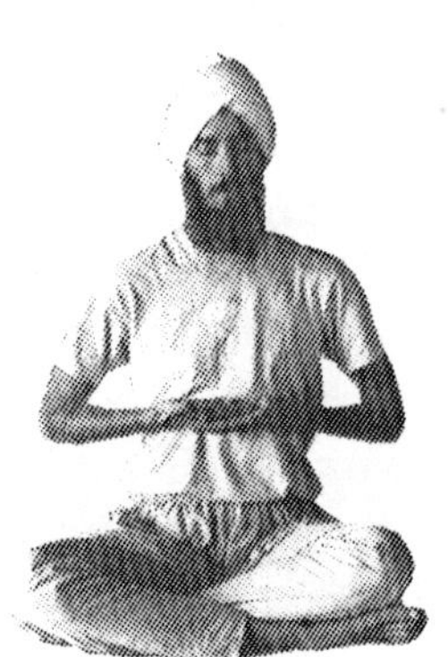

As you chant, slightly pull the navel with each repetition, mentally feeling the navel connect to the spine. This brings a sensitivity of speech and greater connectivity to your words. It purifies the liver energy, sexual energy, and stimulates the fusion (bliss) channel. Move the navel in rhythm with the chant and you may feel a heat build at the navel point. This can be channelled into raising of the Kundalini Prana.

11) Camel ride : 1 to 3 minutes

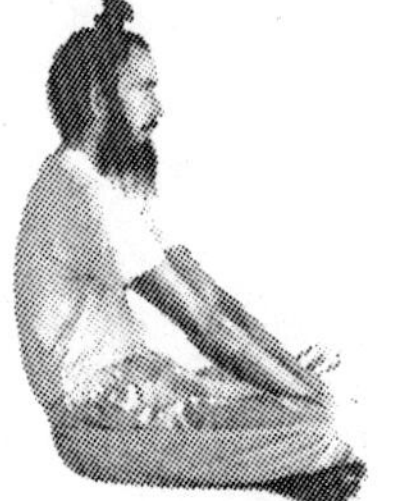

Sitting in easy pose, hands holding onto the shins, flex the lower spine forward as you inhale, back as you exhale. The head remains relatively still. Start slowly and gradually develop a more rapid movement. Mentally direct the breath during the inhale down the front and during each exhale up the spine as you lightly squeeze the perineum. When finished; inhale deeply and hold a Mhul Bhand for thirty seconds.

12) Spinal Twist : 1 to 2 minutes

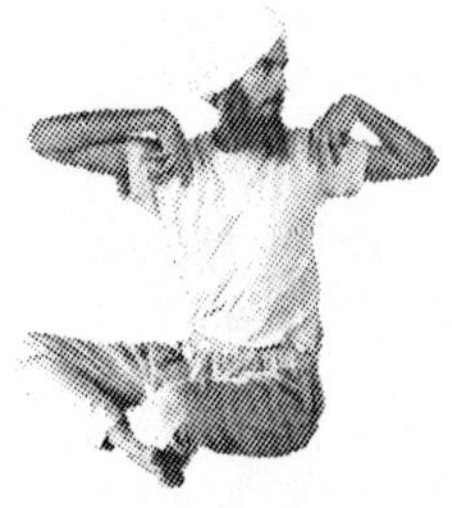

Hands on top of shoulders, elbows out to sides. Inhale as you twist to the left, exhale twisting to the right. As you warm up, increase the pace keeping the movement smooth as you pivot around the spine. When finished inhale and hold a Mhul Bhand for 20 to 30 seconds. Exhale and apply a Maha Bhand for 15 to 30 seconds.

AURIC SET

Remember to keep your navel connection and shoulders relaxed. Apply your full presence (do not let the mind wander) with each movement.

1) Hammer : 3 to 5 minutes

Sit on the heels. Bring the left arm straight in front, palm facing to the right. Extend the right arm with palm also facing to the right. Move right arm underneath the left arm and wrap the fingers of the right hand over the left hand so that the palm of the right hand is against the backside of the left. Then curl the fingers of left hand over the fingers of the right. If this is too difficult; simply interlace the fingers into a fist with arms extended straight out in front.

Inhale the arms 60 degrees above horizontal, exhale 60 degrees below horizontal. Keep the arms straight. Feel yourself vitalizing the body with a perfect symmetry of muscular balance of the two sides of the body. When finished inhale the arms straight up and hold the breath for 15 seconds while applying Mhul Bhand. Exhale, inhale, exhale and apply Maha Bhand for 15 seconds.

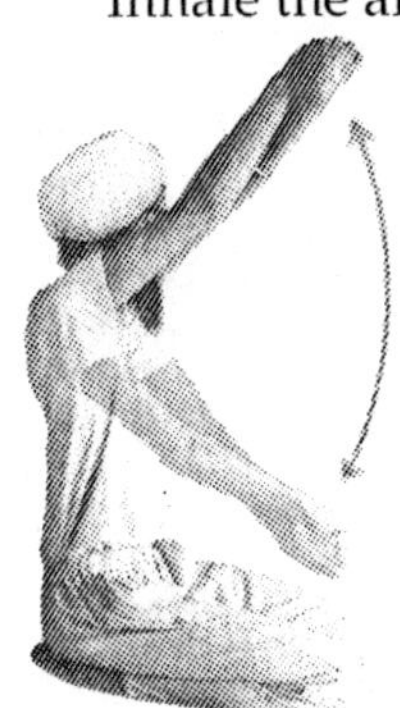

2) Auric Sweep : 3 to 11 minutes

Sit in easy pose. Bring both arms straight out in front with the palms facing each other about four inches apart. Inhale as you sweep the arms back, exhale as you sweep them forwards to original position. Keep the hands stiff and sweep exactly the same path every time in a rhythmical smooth motion. Increase the pace as the breath strengthens. Now here's the secret. Blink the eyes open just as the hands are a few inches apart, looking at the space between the hands, keep the eyes closed the rest of the time. If the mind wanders; mentally chant **"Sat"** on the inhale and **"Naam"** on the exhale.

3) Pushing Walls Apart : 3 to 5 minutes

Hold both arms straight out to the sides, palms facing out. Keep the wrists bent at 90 degrees as if pushing two walls apart, shoulders and face relaxed. Look at the tip of the nose and maintain a long deep relaxed breath. This exercise builds a relationship between the brain and heart. It is a wonderful rejuvenation.

4) Pouring Energy Back and Forth: 3 to 5 minutes.

Left arm straight out to the side, palm facing up. Right arm straight overhead, palm facing in. Keep the angle between the arms 90 degrees as you inhale the left arm straight up and lower the right arm to horizontal, exhale to original position. Keep the hands flat and the motion slow and eloquent as you imagine pouring prana back and forth between the hands. Try extending out through the fingertips into the sky, sweeping a vast area back and forth.

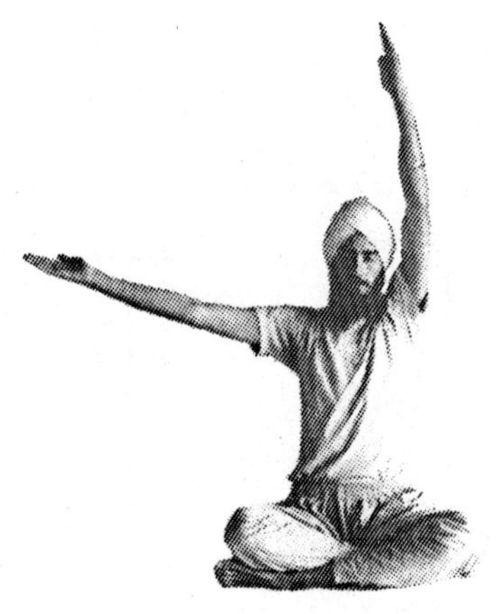

5) Baby Pose : Chant "Ong" : 5 minutes

Sit on the heels. Lower the forehead to the floor and extend the hands in front of you on the floor with the palms flat together. Feel your innocence and simplicity as you chant "**Ong,**" inhaling whenever you need to. Become a vibrating machine, particularly the forehead. Say hello to the crystals under the ground.

6) Either lie on the back for relaxation or sit for meditation.

Rocking to Enlightenment

An easy, not too serious Kriya, that is fun to do in the evening just to get things rolling or to lighten up a bit. Enjoyable with a few friends. Sit in easy pose, as a yogi, serene, jolly, with eyes that have seen great wisdom. The eyes are closed. Hands hold opposite elbows, which are relaxed by the sides.

Pretend that you have been sitting on top of a Himalayan mountain for around 400 years. You have seen lots come and go, and just to pass the time, you start chanting:

"Ha Ha Ha Ha Ri Ri Ri Ri"

Rock from side to side in rhythm with the chant (from side to side on each sound), allowing the breath to adjust by itself. "Ha" is a sound from the navel and provides power. When pronouncing "Ri," make sure the tongue flicks strongly against the upper pallet (pronounced as a hard "r." "Ri" is a sound of intuitive intelligence, as the Rishis might tell you, and the sound is felt from the third eye. The sound "Hari" helps connect the navel and head, regulates the heart, cleans the emotions, and resonates with the dance of creation.

Move back and forth for about ten minutes and hold the breath when finished for not too long.

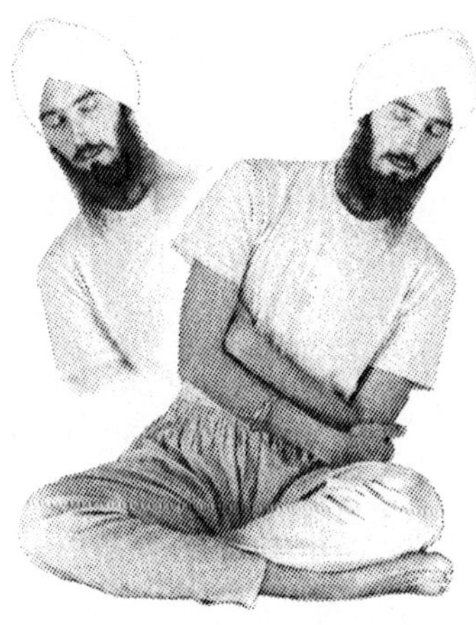

Strengthening the Nervous System

1) Finger Curls : 4 + 1 minutes

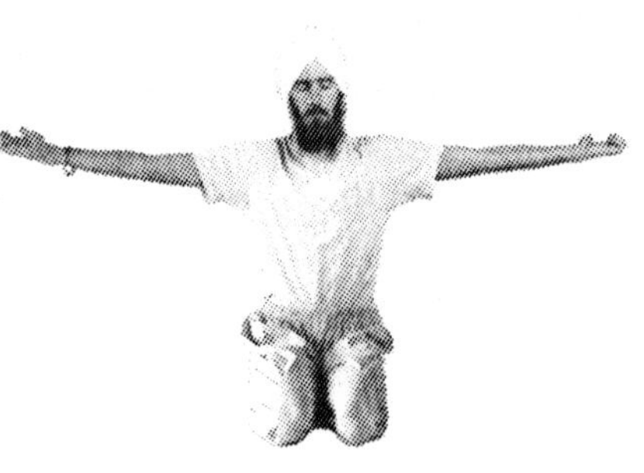

Sitting on the heels or in easy pose extend the arms straight out to sides, horizontal with the floor, palms facing up, thumbs out to sides. Exhale as you curl the fingers into the palms, inhale as you straighten them, with a pace approaching a breath of fire for 4 minutes. Thumbs remain still and pointing back. Then turn palms over (facing down) and continue for 1 minute more. This is a excellent brain exercise.

2) Overhead Arm Crossing : 4 minutes

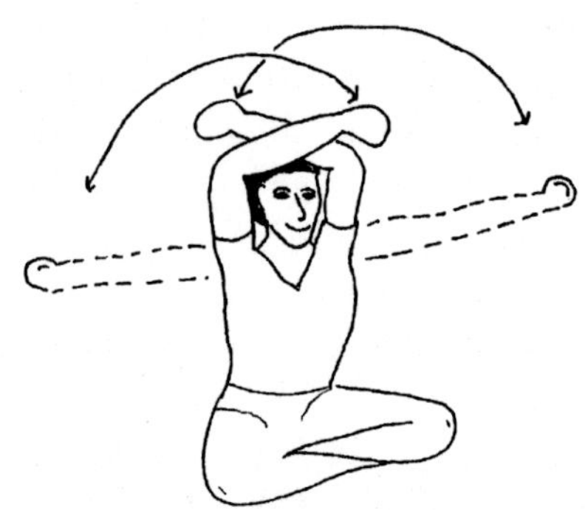

Place the thumbs on the mound of the little fingers and close the hands into fists. Extend arms straight out to the sides. Exhale as you cross the arms overhead, inhale as you bring them out horizontal. Alternate crossing the arms in front and back of head (keeping arms above the head). Develop a powerful breath. This exercise helps to cleanse the Lymph.

3) Super Dynamic Stretch : 4 minutes

Legs straight out in front. Hold the arms straight out in front with palms down. Exhale, bringing the head to the knees, inhale up, **keeping the arms parallel to the floor at all times.** It creates a stretch which helps to align the skeletal structure. Build the pace to a rapid momentum and a powerful breath.

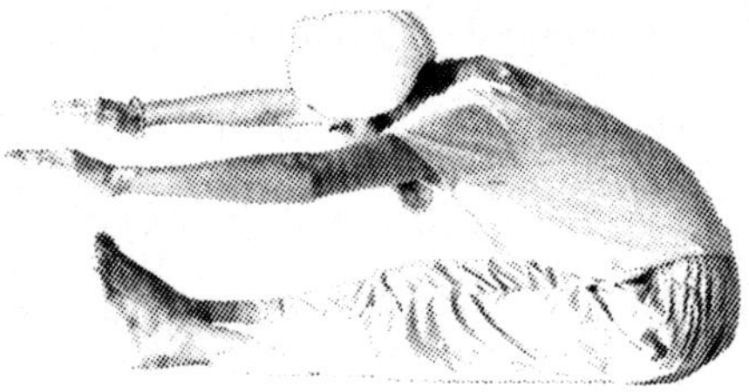

4) Temple-palms Spinal Twist with Legs out : 2 to 3 minutes

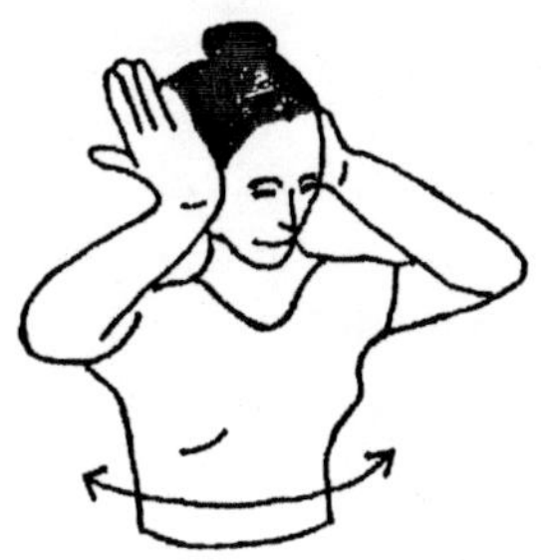

Legs remaining straight on the floor, place the palms against the temples. Thumbs remain separate and point back. Thumb and fingers are stiff and do not rest against the head. Inhale as you twist to the left, exhale as you twist to the right, building to a rapid smooth movement. Keep the palms pressed against the temples.

5) Broken breath Bowing with Legs out: 2 to 3 minutes

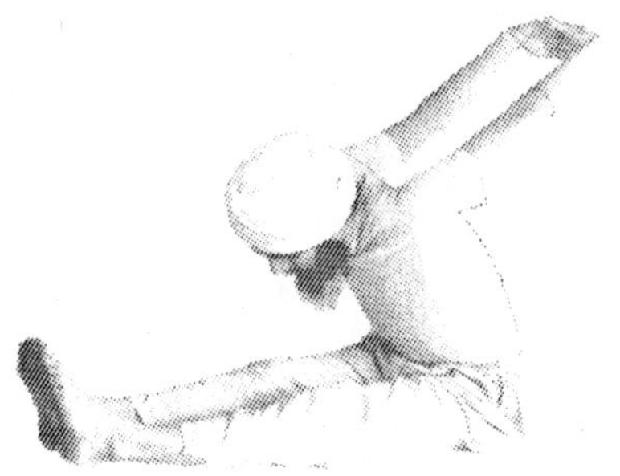

Legs remaining out, clasp the hands together behind the back. Inhale in four distinct parts as you lower the head to the knees and raise the arms as high as you can. Exhale as you return to the original position.

6) Horse Stance broken breath Bowing : 3 to 5 minutes

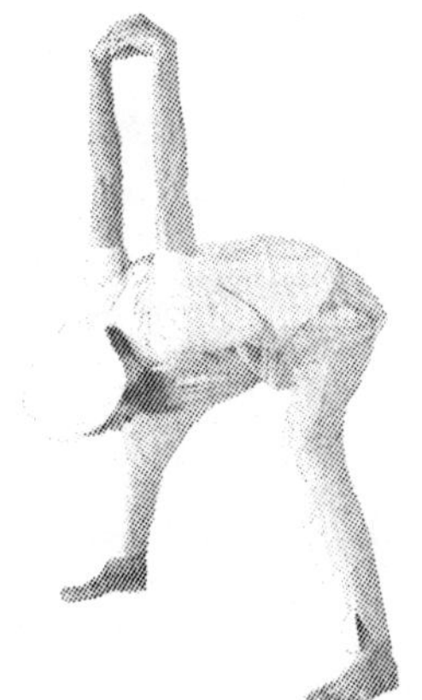

Stand up into horse stance, feet 2 to 3 feet apart, bend at the knees. Same motion as in previous exercise. Inhaling and lowering the head in 4 parts as you raise the arms up behind the back, exhale to standing position. Keep the knees bent throughout.

6b) Horse Stance : 3 to 5 minutes (Optional)

Stand in horse stance, holding opposite elbows (arms relaxed against torso). Long deep breathing. Sink down as if sitting in a chair while keeping the spine straight.

7) Dynamic Life Nerve Stretch (one leg): 3 minutes each side.

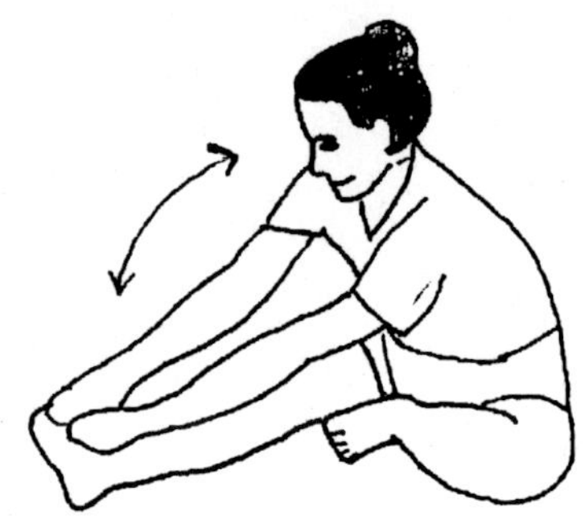

Sit down with the left leg straight and tuck the heel of the right foot against the groin. Keeping the leg straight, hold the big toe. Exhale as you lower the head to the knee, inhale up and tilt head back *slightly*. Develop a rapid mechanical motion with strong breathing as you surrender into the exercise. 3 minutes, then switch legs and repeat.

8a) Jumping Bean : 2 minutes

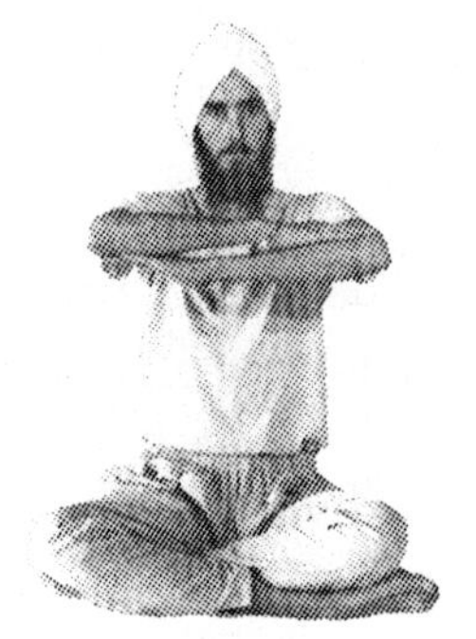

Sit in easy pose. Hold opposite elbows with the hands, and hold the arms horizontal. Rock forward slightly as you inhale and jump the body up, like a jumping bean. Continue hopping up and down. *(Only do this if your body is fit for it).*

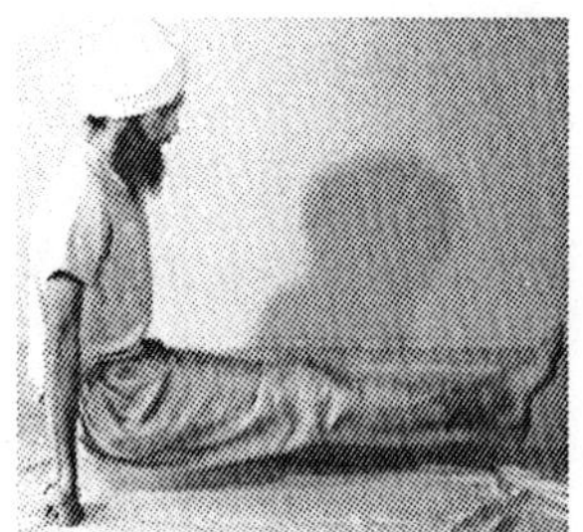

8b) Body Drops : 26 or 54 times

Quickly stretch legs out, hands or fist on floor by sides. Lift the body up, and drop it.

8c) Jumping Bean (as in 8a): 1 more minute

The secret is a positive attitude and drawing your energy up, in a sense of joyful lightness. This exercise will make you sweat, eliminates depression (just try to be depressed after this!), and is fun.

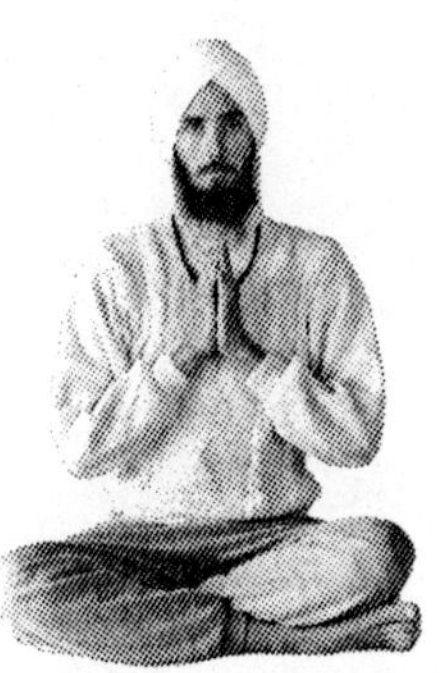

9) Long Deep Breathing: 5 to 10 minutes

Palms together in prayer pose at the heart. Long deep peaceful breathing.

A Fun Pick Me Up

Sit straight and either:

- Rest hands on the knees in Gyan mudra (thumbs and index finger touching).
- Or Bring arms straight out to each side with palms facing up.

Inhale in four equal segments (deep and rapid) in the following manner:

Inhale as you turn the head to the left, inhale as you turn the head to the right, inhale as you turn the head to the left, inhale as you turn the head to the right.

Face center and exhale as you chant the following **twice** in a quick and very spirited tempo:

"Wahe Guru Wahe Guru
Wahe Wahe Wahe Guru"

Pronounced: *Wha-hay Guroo*

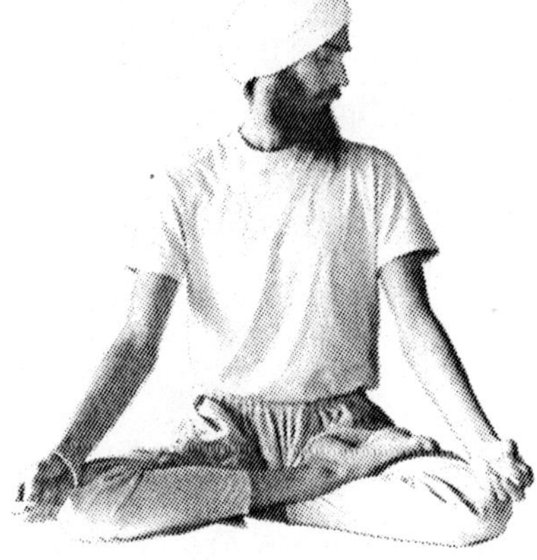

A Different Kind of Bowing

Sit with a straight spine and relaxed shoulders. Hands are in front of the chest at shoulder level with both palms facing forwards, the right palm touching the back of the left palm. Chant in a meditative monotone :

"Har Guru, Siri Guru, Wahe Guru"

for a minute to establish the sound current. Then as "**Har Guru**" is chanted lean forward 1/3 of the way to the ground. As "**Siri Guru**" is chanted lean forwards 2/3 of the way, and as "**Wahe Guru**" is chanted lower all the way to the floor (staying in the mudra), then quickly rise to the original position and continue in this way, maintaining the grace and power of the **rhythm for 11 minutes.**

Then stay down, hands still in the proper mudra, and begin a **Breath of Fire for 2 or 3 minutes**. Relax for a few moments and come out of posture, meditate silently, becoming inwardly conscious of the field of awareness in which you sit and observe.

Hari is creative force. *Guru* is transmitting power of your higher presence. *Siri* is an inner expansion and *Wahe* is ecstatic bliss. Thus this mantra is about creating the expansion to awaken the bliss of one's deeper self.

Pronunciation:

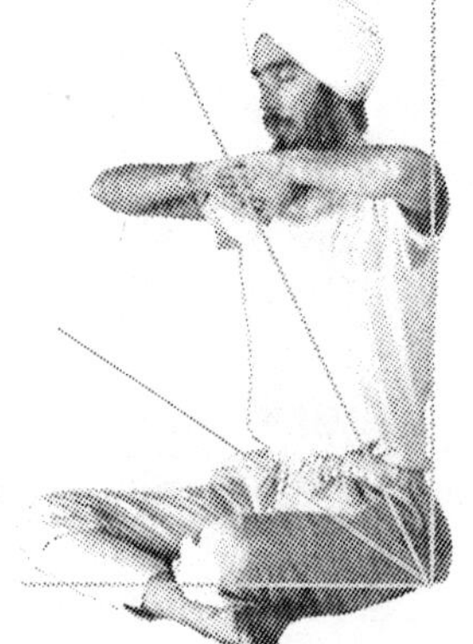

"Har" the "a" is short and rhythms with "u" of udder, "r" sounds as a cross between an "r" and a "d." The tongue flicks against the upper palate to sound it. As the tongue leaves the palette, a slight "i" sound trails.

"Siri" rhythms with "city"

"Wahe" Wha-hay, "Wha!" is given emphasis of an uprising tone, indicating excitement, or an ecstatic mood.

"Guru" Guroo

Relax on back. Feel your body sink into the earth. Come back light and rejuvenated.

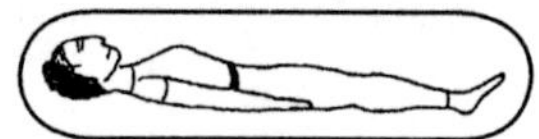

A Little Bit of Movement

Do a few stretches and this exercise to loosen up a bit before sitting. Particularly good for the evening.

Sit on the heels and do the following movement with a full breath, **flowing smoothly from one part to the next.**

Clasp hands (fingers interlaced) behind the back, inhale as you lower the forehead to the ground while raising the arms as high as possible behind the back, exhale as you return to original position and bring the arms straight in front of you (palms do not touch), inhale as you sweep the arms back while rising up on the knees, exhale as you sit back down, inhale as you bring the arms straight overhead (palms together), exhale the arms down and clasp them behind the back to continue the cycle.

The entire sequence is as one movement.

Time: Whatever you feel like.

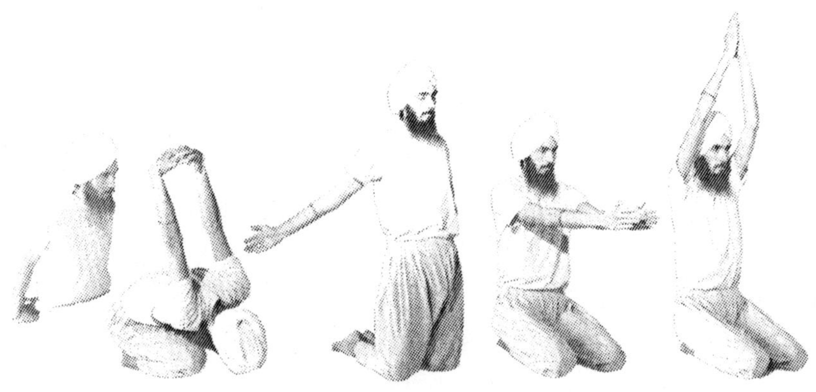

This practice originated in a dream in which I was teaching it to about a thousand people in a gathering, to create the space for a meditative transmission.

Lymph, Blood, Liver, & Maintenance Set

A great set for both beginning and experienced practitioners. Adjust times to your capacity.

1) Sit in celibate pose (in-between the heels). 7 minutes.

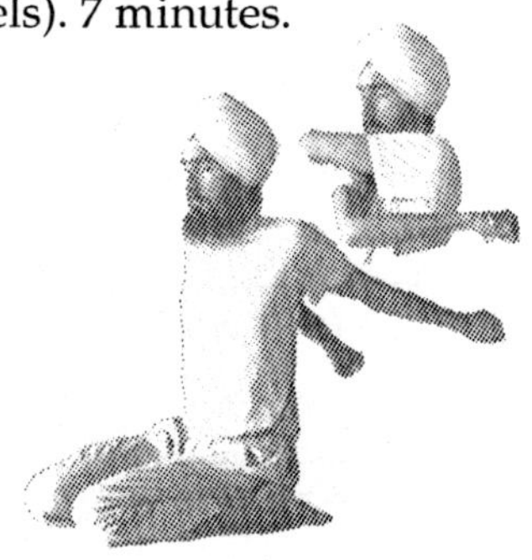

Place the thumbs on the mound of the small finger and form the hands into fists over the thumbs. Inhale as you sweep the arms back, exhale as the arms cross in front of you. Shoulders remain relaxed and arms horizontal. This exercise cleanses the lymph glands and develop endurance.

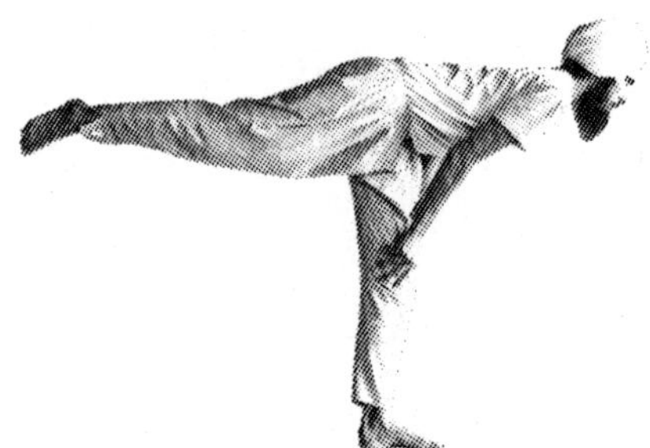

2) Stand horizontal on one leg : 2 to 3 minutes on each leg.

Bend at the waist so the body and opposite leg is horizontal. The hands are used as a brace just above the knee. Keep the body straight.

3a) Modified shoulder stand : 1 to 3 minutes

Using the hands to brace the lower back. Bend at the knees, so the feet are at the buttocks. Keep the knees stretched up to the sky (this is the secret).

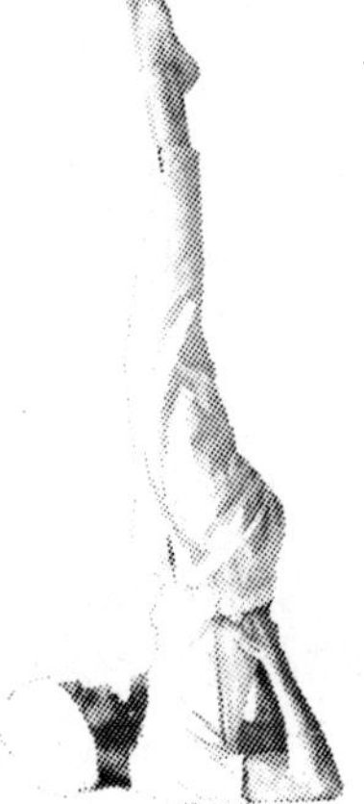

3b) Inhale as the legs are straightened, exhale as you return the feet to the original position. As you exhale make a humming sound that is like a sigh of relief. 2 to 3 minutes.

3c) Rest on the back : 2 or 3 minutes.

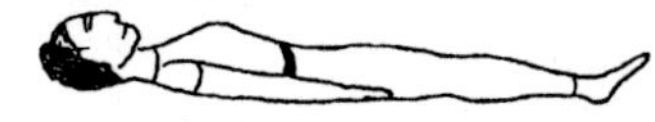

4) Spinal Twist : 2 to 5 minutes

Sit on the heels, arms stretched straight overhead, palms flat together. Inhale as you twist to the left, exhale twisting to the right as you pivot around the spine. Continue at a moderate to rapid pace. If the arms want to bend or come down, keep them straight, as this will build the vitality and magnetic field of the upper centers. Powerful breath. When finished, keep the arms up and move directly to the next exercise.

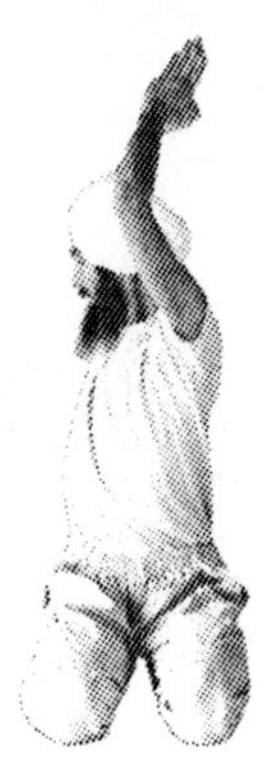

5) Side to Side Sway:

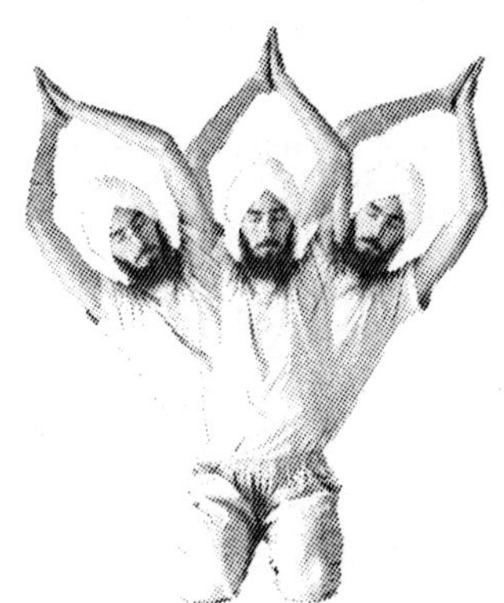

2 to 5 minutes.

Keep the arms up and palms flat together. Inhale as you bend sideways to the left, exhale as you bend to the right, like a tree swaying in the wind. Keep the arms straight. Feel your harmony. This is excellent for cleansing the liver.

6) Alternate Leg Lifts : 3 to 7 minutes

Lie on the back and lift one leg at a time to 90 degrees and back down again. Touch the floor gently, and keep the lower back firmly on the floor. When finished inhale both legs up and hold with long deep breathing for 1 or 2 minutes.

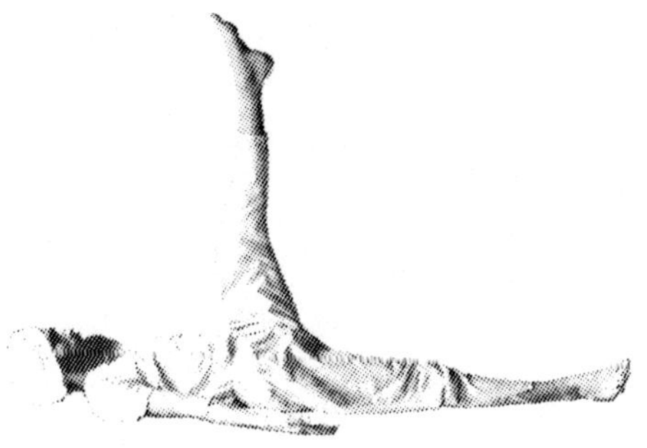

7) Left leg straight on floor in front, heel of right foot against the groin.

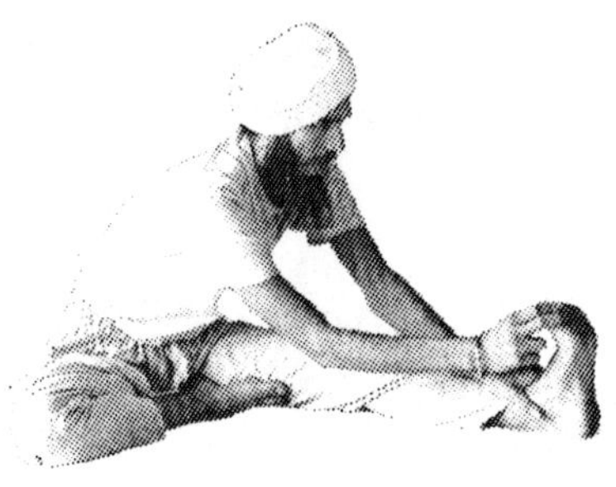

With the right hand grip the big toe of the left foot and with the thumb press against the toenail and with the index finger press against the back of the toe opposite the toenail (this stimulates the pituitary gland). The other hand may hold onto the ankle. Arms straight, back straight, and fix the eyes on the tip of the big toe and do not move your focus an inch. Stick the tongue out and keep it stretched out for the duration of the exercise. **Begin an exaggerated panting breath, like a dog for 7 minutes.**

Cleans the blood, increases the digestive fire, helps to release and clear cellular memory, and makes the eyes strong. The secret is in keeping the eyes absolutely focused on a 1/4 square inch area at the tip of the toe, not wavering for a second.

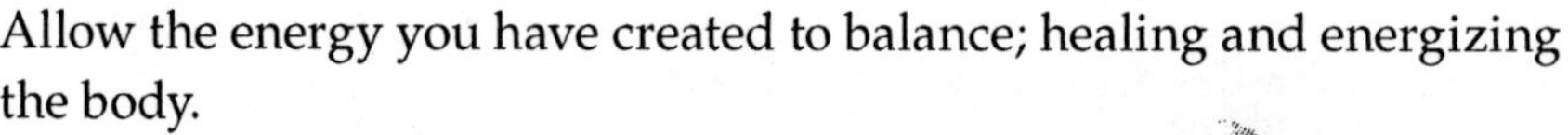

8) Relax for 10 to 15 minutes.

Allow the energy you have created to balance; healing and energizing the body.

9) Meditate

The Invincible Four U's

These simple postures align the subtle and physical energy bodies, thereby helping to overcome weaknesses of many kinds. Do each one for up to eleven minutes, with a one or two minute rest in between (lying on the back).

Keep a full deep easy breath going throughout each exercise, using the breath to help your mind stay present in the posture. As you become more adept, pay particular attention to opening the spine. Feel energy coming in through the legs and arms, mixing in the lower and mid-spinal region and then flowing throughout the body, so that it feels whole and connected. At times apply a mhula bhanda. **Keep the posture as still as possible.**

After a few weeks or months of practice, forget about the breath and instead focus on keeping the posture as still as possible, while the mind continues to draw energy in through the limbs as before. Do not move a muscle. This transfers awareness to the subtle energy aspect of your body, whereby you can quicken, smooth and refine energy with your mind. Spiral the energy deep into the bones.

1) Lie on the back with arms and legs pointing straight up, feeling their subtle extension into the sky. In particular, draw this cosmic energy through the legs into the lower back. Relax any tension in the body, feet separate, shoulders relaxed.

2) Lift the legs up and over your head, so that they are parallel to the ground. The arms are also extended flat on the ground behind your head.

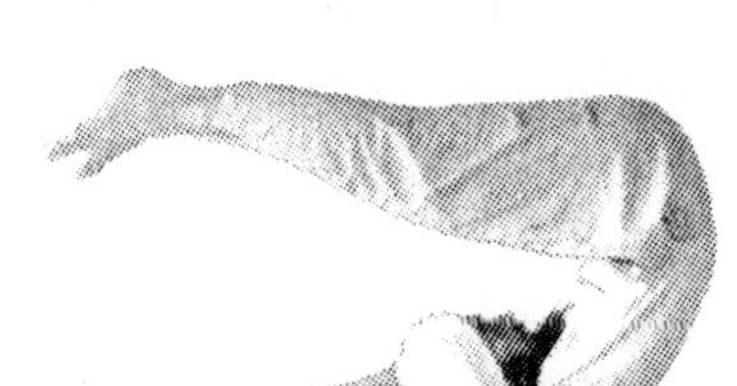

3) Sit up with legs straight in front of you, arms straight (parallel to ground).

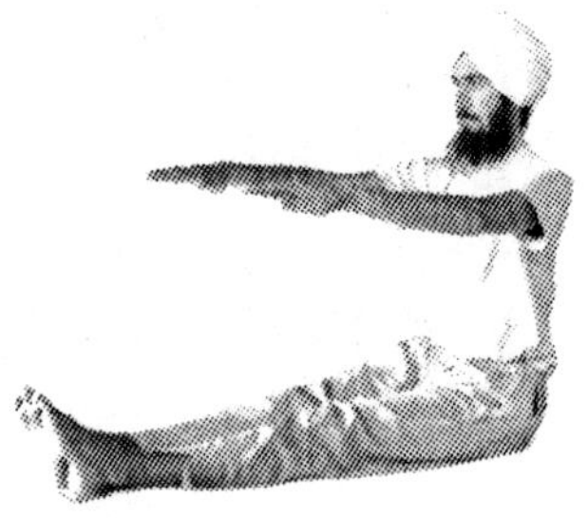

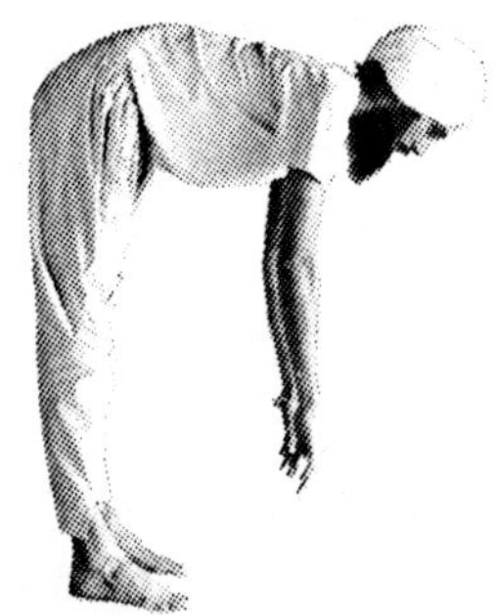

4) Stand up, bend ninety degrees at the waist and let the arms hang straight down. Concentrate on opening the spine, starting from the tailbone, open and vital. Spread the shoulders apart, so there is a feeling of opening in the upper chest. Shaking in the muscles is a cleansing of toxins and the nerve channels.

For the full benefit, these postures are to be held perfectly still. Pain will come, let it burn out. This practice brings the ability to do with less sleep and food while giving maximum output. It regenerates the body from its burdens, helps release the charge and blockages of past cellular memory while clearing the meridians. Excellent for the lower back.

<u>**Variations**</u>

- **Long Deep Breathing**
- **Breath of Fire :** Clears blockages and energizes.
- **Relaxed, almost still breathing :** This is good after initial blockages have been cleared in previous practice. Perfect the posture, holding absolutely still, remaining for the full 11 minutes. Holding absolutely still with presence sensitizes the pranic body. You can then absorb and circulated very refined pranas through the direction of the mind, to bring a deep rest and healing.
- **Chanting :** Provided you stay very present, gives extra will and focus to work through any blocks. Helps establish a relationship with the mantra.

A General Workout

1) Bowing : 3 to 5 minutes

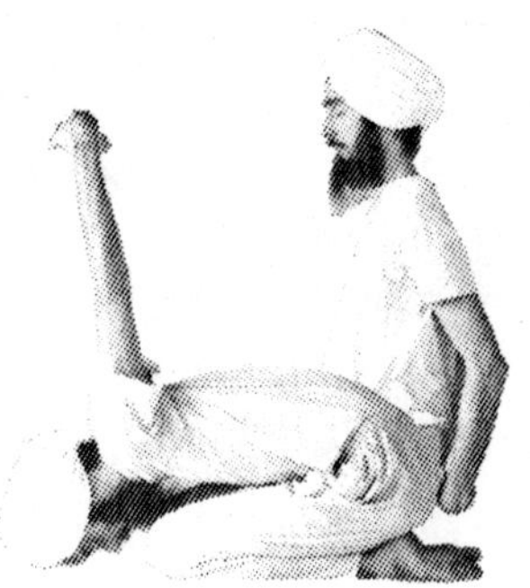

Sit on the heels and interlace the hands into a fist behind the back. Inhale as you lower the forehead to the floor while raising the arms up as high as possible, exhale to original position. Moderate to rapid pace with a smooth rhythm and strong breath.

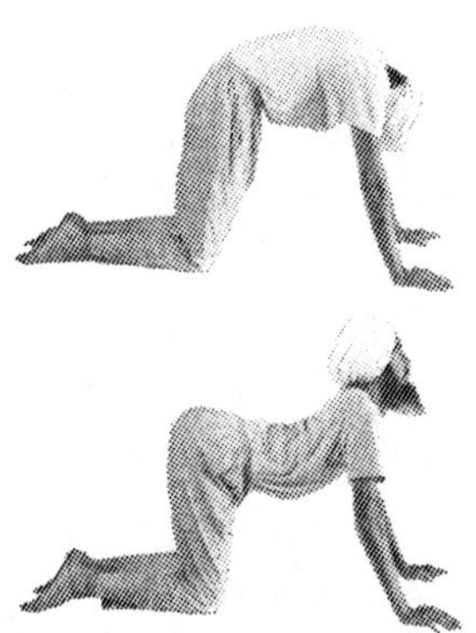

2) Cat/Cow Flex : 1 minute

Come on to the hands and knees. Flex the spine, inhaling as the spine flexes down and the head up. Exhale as the spine flexes up and the head down.

3) Dynamic Tiger : 2 minutes each leg

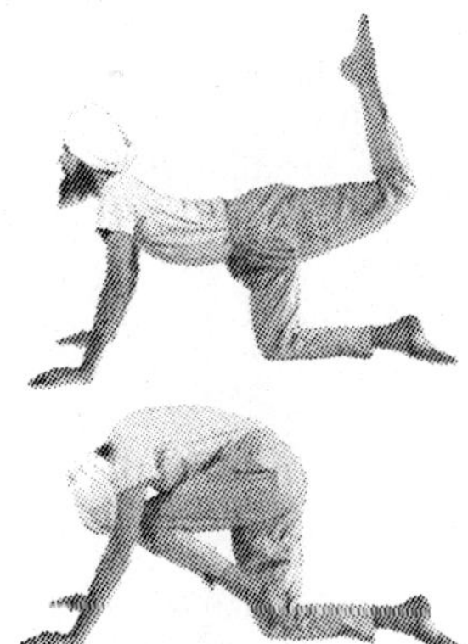

In the same posture, inhale as the left leg swings up and back, spine flexes down, and head up. Exhale as the leg moves in, spine flexes up, and head down, so that the knee almost touches the forehead. Increase to a rapid pace, with powerful breathing as you warm into the exercise.

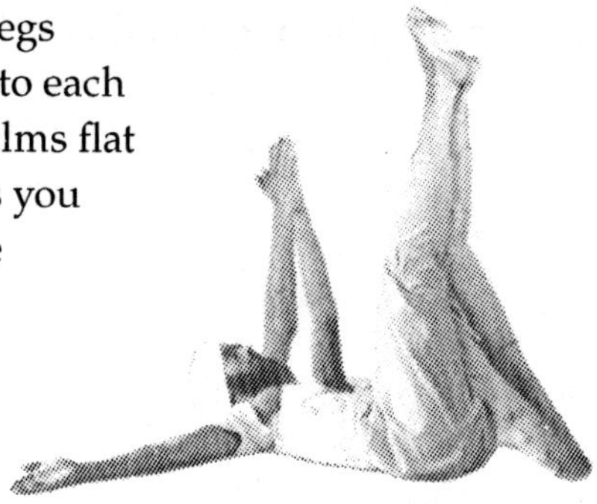

4) Lying on the back, bring the legs straight up. Arms are straight out to each side, an inch above the ground. Palms flat and stiff, but not tensed. Exhale as you bend the legs so that the feet come down to the buttocks and at the same time sweep the arms up so that the palms are four inches apart. Inhale as you lower the arms and raise the legs straight. Move in a moderate rhythm, smooth, and with a strong full breath. 3 to 11 minutes.

Use the navel energy to move the limbs. The moving legs generate energy in the lower back which is brought up the spine and distributed by the sweeping arms. The whole coordinated movement helps harmonize the body and relax the brain.

5) Leg lifts (both legs) : 1 to 4 minutes

Remaining on the back, inhale as you lift both legs up to 90 degrees, exhale down touching the heels lightly to the ground. Keep the legs straight.

If your lower back raises excessively from the ground, then lift to one leg at a time until you build the strength to lift both legs while keeping the lower back pressed against the floor. You want to reinforce the correct muscle patterns.

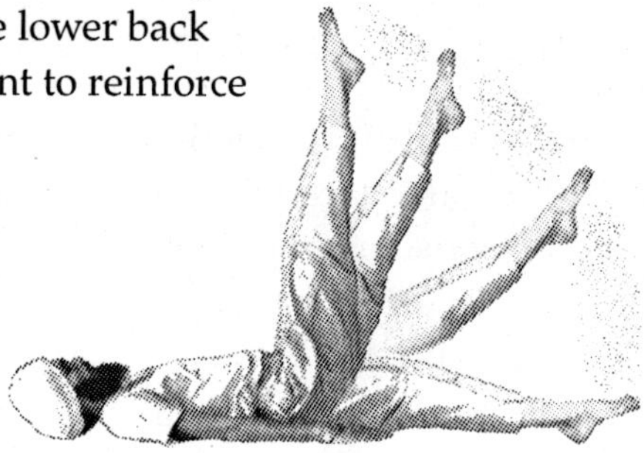

6) Dynamic Cobra : 1 to 3 minutes or 108 times

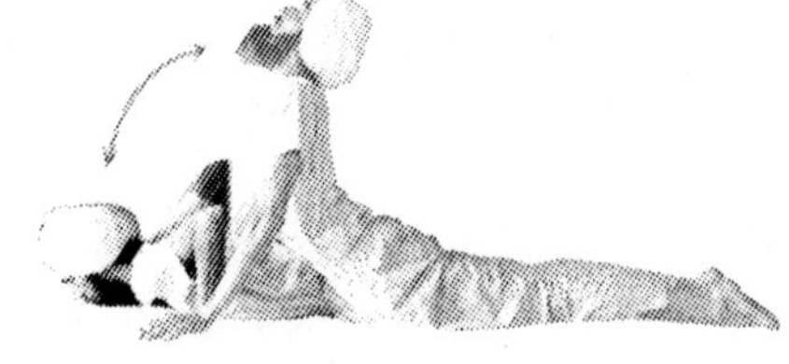

Lying on the stomach bring the hands flat on the ground by the shoulders. Heels remain together. Inhale as you push up and arch the entire spine, hips remaining on the ground. Exhale down. Develop a steady rhythm and increase the speed for the last half of the exercise. As you are arched in the up position look to the third eye and squeeze the buttocks and perineum to move energy through the tailbone and up the spine.

7) Arm lifts : Ground to overhead : 1 to 4 minutes

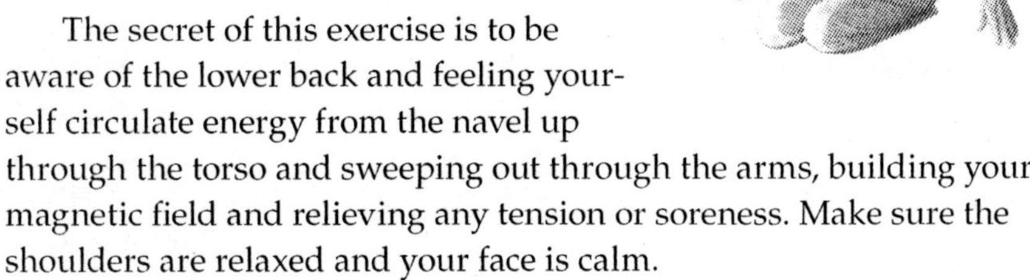

Sit on the heels. Breathe deeply a few times to fill out your energy in the lower back. Inhale the arms up so that the palms lightly touch overhead, exhale as you lower the arms and rotate them so that the palms face down as the fingertips lightly touch the ground. As the arms are inhaled up again rotate the arms so that the palms face each other as thy touch overhead.

The secret of this exercise is to be aware of the lower back and feeling yourself circulate energy from the navel up through the torso and sweeping out through the arms, building your magnetic field and relieving any tension or soreness. Make sure the shoulders are relaxed and your face is calm.

8) Kundalini Lotus

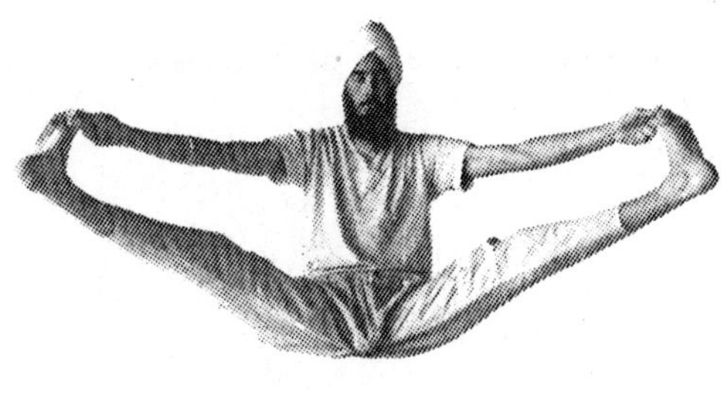

Balance on the tail bone as you lift the legs straight, grabbing the toes. Press the tips of each toe with the thumbs, thereby stimulating the head centers. Spread the legs wide and hold with long deep breathing for 1 to 3 minutes. Then for 1 minute exhale as you bring the legs together and inhale as you move them apart.

9) Frogs : 54 or 108 times

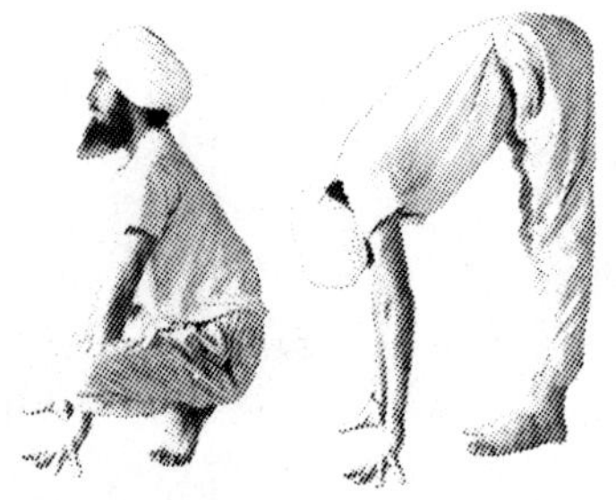

Squat with the heels together and off the ground. The feet are angled towards each side, fingertips resting on the ground in front of you, and head looking forward. Inhale as you straighten the legs, fingertips remaining on the ground, heels remain together and touch the ground. Exhale down to original position. Maintain awareness of the spine throughout the exercise while breathing deep and powerfully.

10) Bowing : 1 to 3 minutes

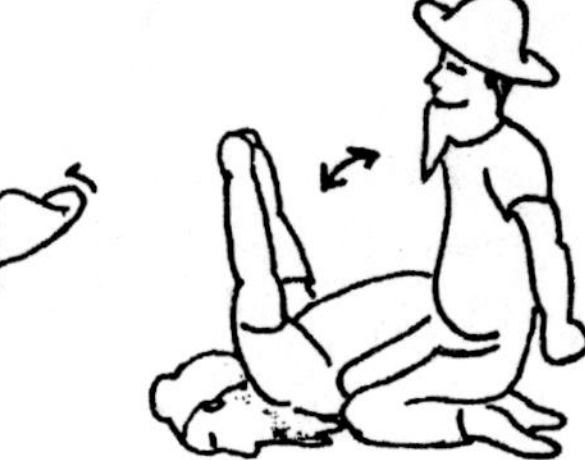

Repeat exercise #1, maintaining a symmetry of each side of the body around your centerline.

11) Relax on the Back

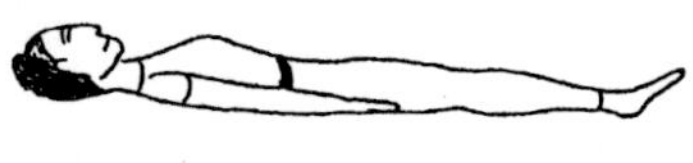

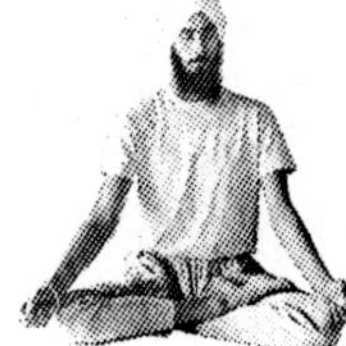

12) Meditate!

Opening the Throat and Adjusting the Metabolism

These exercises are best done in silence with strong connected breathing, dissolving the mind into the motion and breath. This set opens the throat, harmonizes body rhythms and strengthens the etheric aspect of the physical body. When we disassociate from our body temple, then our etheric body is ungrounded and our thoughts are not restful or coherent with our environment.

Warm up first, particularly the hips and lower spine. A suggestion is to move around a bit (running in place, kicks, dancing..), then Bridge pose for 3 minutes, then a few spinal flex exercises.

1) **Sitting on the heels,** extend both arms straight out to the sides with palms facing down. In a smooth and rapid rhythm inhale as you turn the head to the left while mentally chanting "Sat," exhale as you turn the head to the right mentally sounding "Naam." **3 Minutes.**

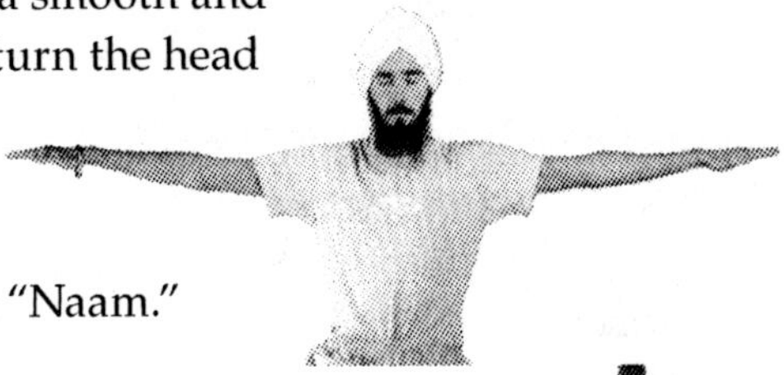

2) **Raise alternate shoulders to the ears.** Inhale a shoulder up, exhale down, inhale the other shoulder up... 1 Minute.

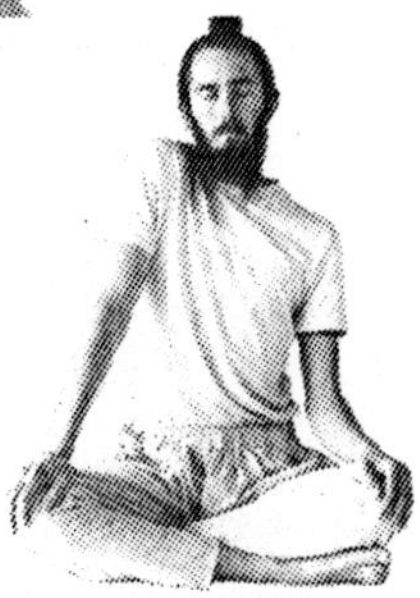

3) **Remaining on the heels with a straight spine,** extend both arms straight in front of you. The palms are facing up and cupped with the sides of the palms touching each other. Feel as if you are receiving a divine gift of nectar. Tilt the head back, keeping the spine straight, and begin a *Breath of Fire*. You may experience a **tightness in the upper chest as the glands begin to secrete. Keep breathing and mix these elixirs into the body.** 3 Minutes.

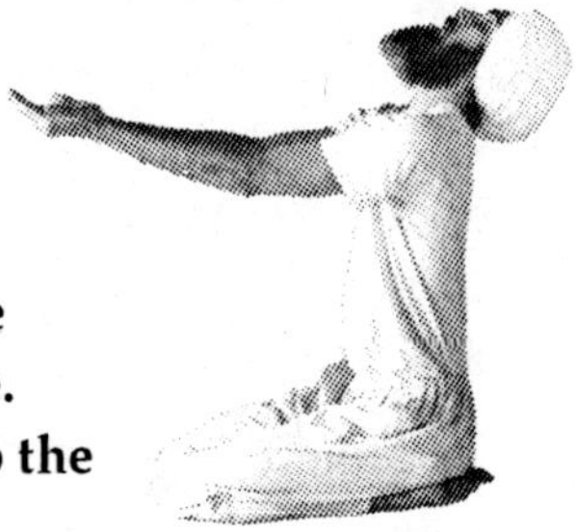

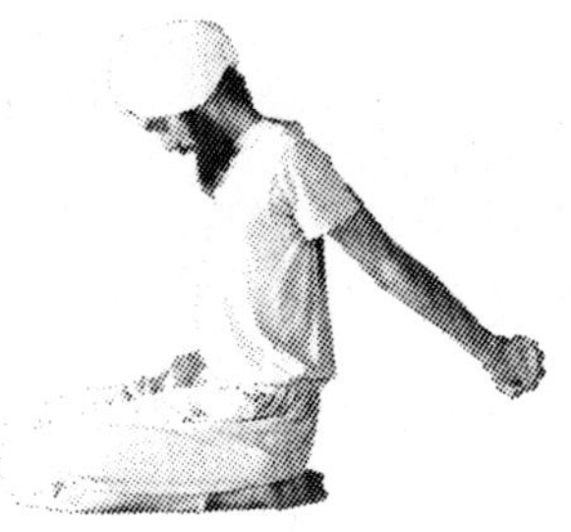

4) **Slowly straighten the head** and relax the arms. Then bring the arms behind the back, fingers interlaced into a fist, and raise the arms as high as possible, keeping the spine straight. Lower the chin to the chest and begin a *Breath of Fire.* **3 Minutes.**

5) **Sit in easy or lotus pose.**

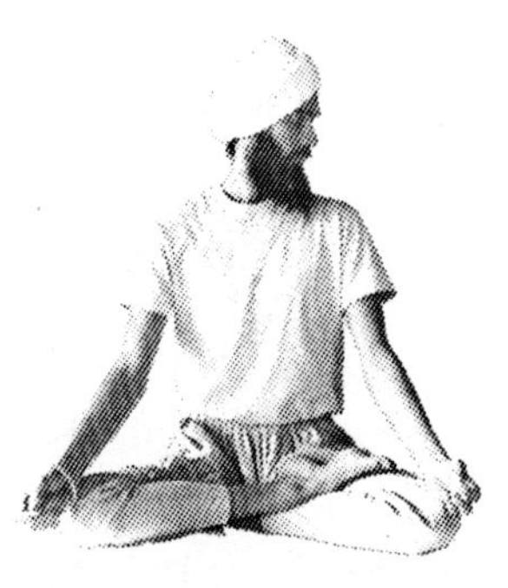

Hands in Gyan mudra (thumb and first finger touch) resting on the knees. Back straight, sit light. Feel yourself as a Yogi, that has watched the ages come and go, sitting on a mountain top for 400 years, you look at the tip of your nose, and inhale as you *slowly* move the head to the left while mentally hearing the sound *"Sat."* Exhale as you *slowly* turn the head to the right while hearing the sound *"Naam."* Watch the world go by the tip of the nose. Hear these sounds fill the sky, and become the sky. Let the nectar drip within of the bliss of just being. Remember to move the head very slowly. **Twenty Six breaths.**

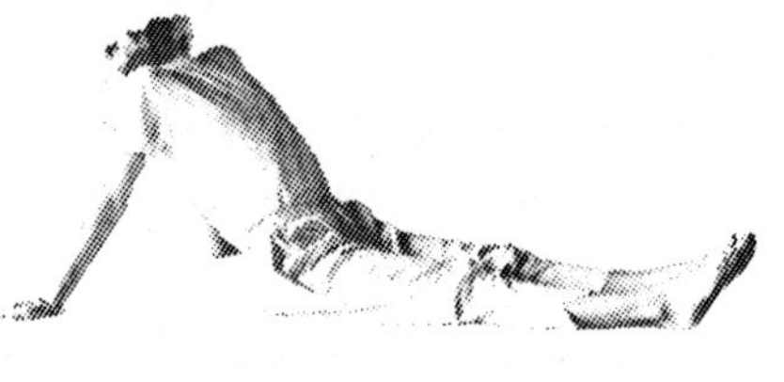

6) **Extend your legs straight out in front.** Lean back and support yourself with your hands. Let the head fall back and remain in this position with a normal breath. There is nothing you have to do, except remain in this position. Close the eyes, or look at a point on the ceiling. You are causing the parathyroid to secret, which means that you will rest deeply and rebalance your chemistry. **After five minutes,** inhale deep, exhale a big sigh as you relax on your back. Cover yourself, and go into a total relaxation for at least ten minutes. Allow the body to balance itself, as you sink deep within the Earth.

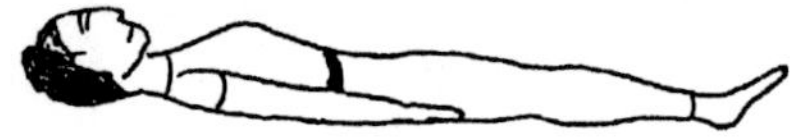

Peaceful Potency

1) Archer Pose, Tongue out : 5 to 11 minutes each side

Back leg straight, front knee over foot. Navel faces forward, hips are tucked in, spine is straight. Feet as shown in illustration.

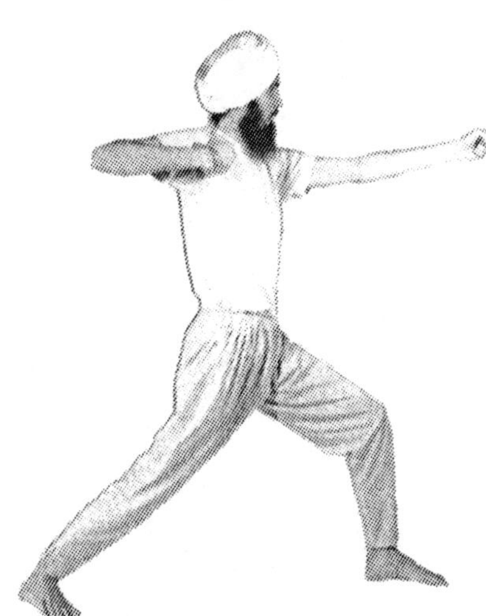

Pretend that you are drawing a bow with the arms, and hold the arms still in this position. Look straight ahead over the fist of the extended arm. Stick the tongue out and keep it stretched. Maintain a powerful exaggerated breath. Do not bounce and let the thighs burn through any resistance.

2a) Relax in Childs Pose : 2 to 3 minutes

Sit on the heels and lower the forehead to the ground in childlike simplicity and innocence.

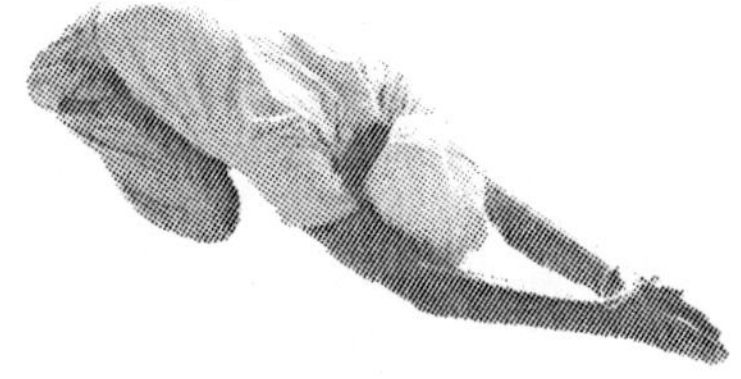

2b) Relax on back : 2 to 3 minutes

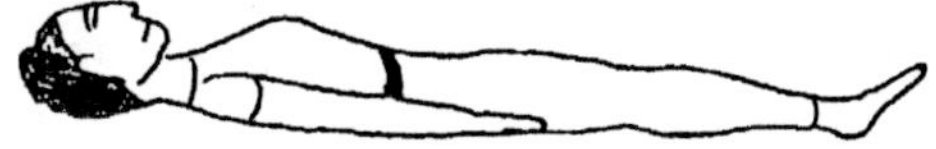

3) Tree Pose, hands on ground : 5 to 11 minutes each side.

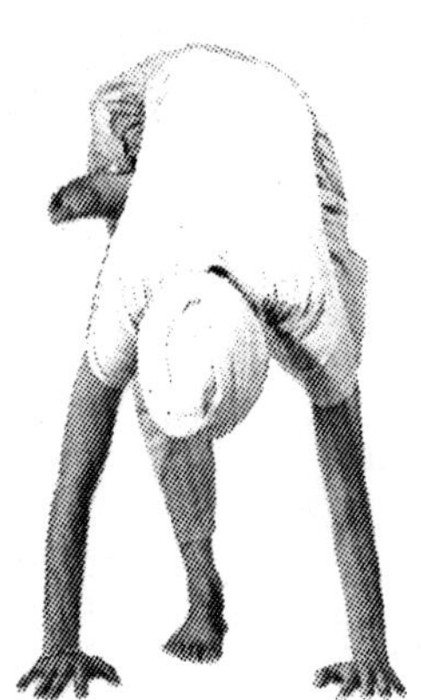

Stand on one leg. Tuck the foot of the opposite leg against the upper thigh of the standing leg. Bend forward and place the palms of the hands flat on the ground. Look down into the ground.

Helps to increase and transmute sexual energy.

4) Lie on back, arms resting by sides.

Lift buttocks off ground as high as possible, with weight on feet and upper back.
2 to 4 minutes.

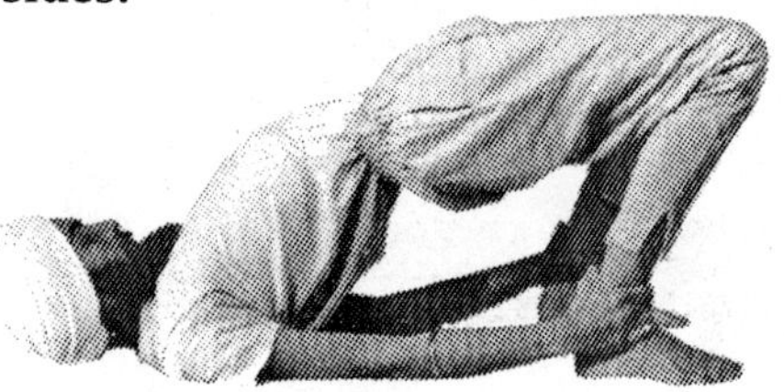

5) Relax on back for 5 to 15 minutes.

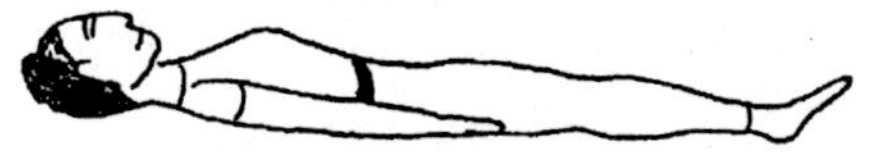

6) Mediation - Sa Ta Na Ma Kriya

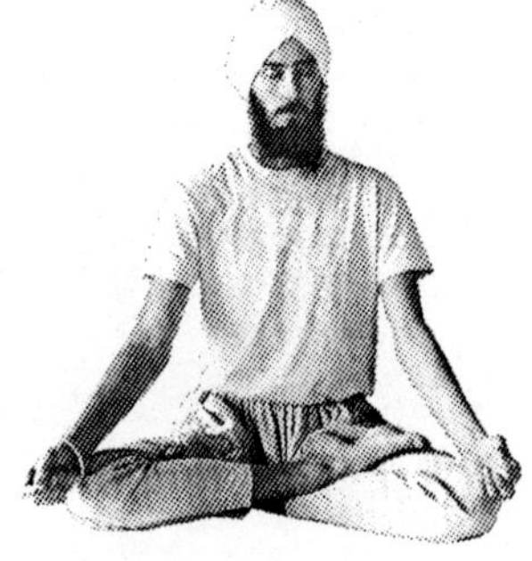

As given on page 104.

Opening Up the Spine

These exercises warm up the spine and prepare the body for meditation. You may want to meditate for a minute or two between exercises. Throughout the set, mentally sound "Sat" as you inhale and "Naam" as you exhale. The set may be shortened by omitting some of the exercises. **This is a good beginning set.**

1a) Slap the back of the hands rapidly against each other.
1 to 2 Minutes.

1b) Slap the forearms of each arm with opposite hands.
1 to 2 Minutes.

1c) Lean forward and slap the lower back in a spirited fashion.
1 Minute.

2) Up and Around : 1 to 3 Minutes

Stand with feet several feet apart. Interlace both hands together in a fist. To start, bend over with the arms hanging down, inhale as you come up sweeping the arms up and over the head, and exhaling as you come down in a full circle. Then reverse directions and continue. Big smooth arcs, deep breath. Opens up the diaphragm.

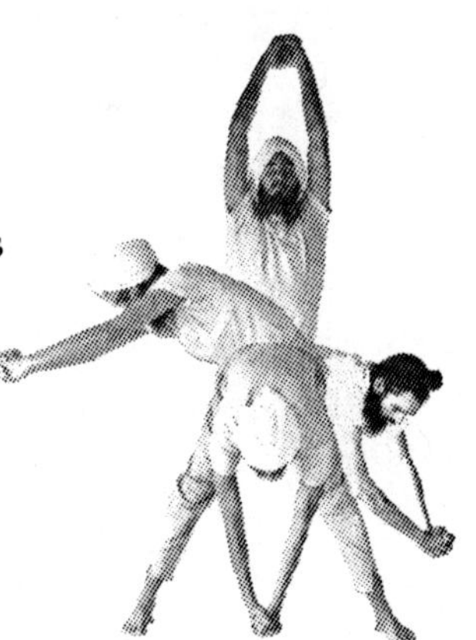

3) Chair Pose :
1 to 3 Minutes : Breath of Fire

Legs several feet apart, squat down and grasp the inside of the ankles with the arms on the inside of the legs. Keep the back horizontal and look forward.

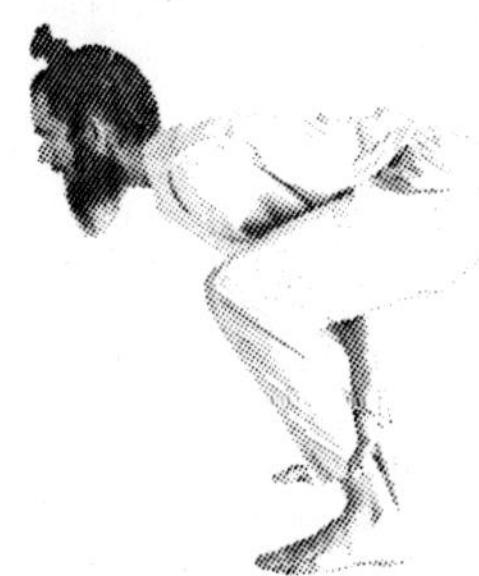

4) Dynamic Life Nerve Stretch : 3 Minutes

Sit on the floor with legs straight out in front and hold onto the toes, or as far as you can stretch while keeping the legs straight. Inhale up, exhale down. Let the head bend back as you come up, so as to prevent any strain on the neck. Move with a deep breath, quickening the pace as you warm up. When finished, inhale up, exhale down. Stay down, inhaling a very deep breath and hold for 15 to 20 seconds while staying very still.

During the exercise become machine like, up and down, totally surrendering into the exercise. Let the mind dissolve on the breath. When we are totally present in an exercise, then we align the etheric body into the physical and recharge ourselves.

5) Camel Ride : 1 to 3 Minutes

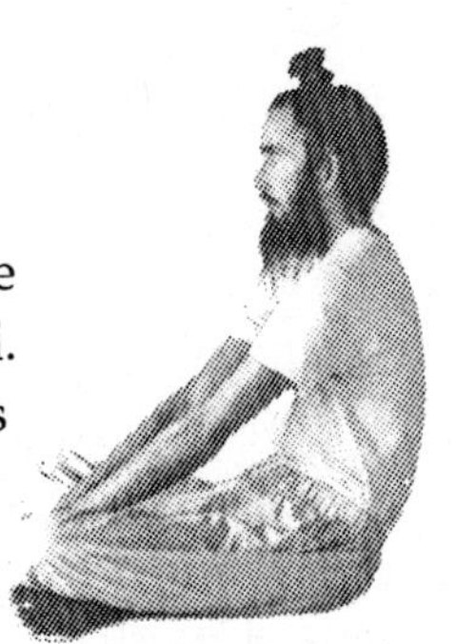

Sit cross-legged and hold the shins. Inhale as you flex the spine forward, exhale as you flex back. The head remains relatively still and shoulders relaxed. When finished hold the breath for 15 to 30 seconds and apply Mhula Bhand. Then breathe deeply for a minute or two focusing between the eyes with a straight back.

6) Spinal Twist : 1 to 3 Minutes

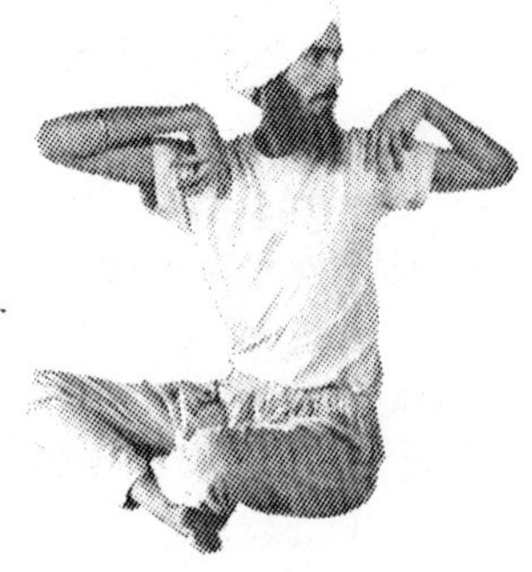

Remaining in easy pose rest the hands on the shoulders, elbows out to the sides. Inhale as you twist the upper body to the left, exhale as you twist to the right. Develop a rapid fluid rhythm. Feel that you are pivoting around the spine. When finished, apply Mhula Bhand with the breath retained.

7) Heart Beargrip Twirl : 1 to 2 Minutes

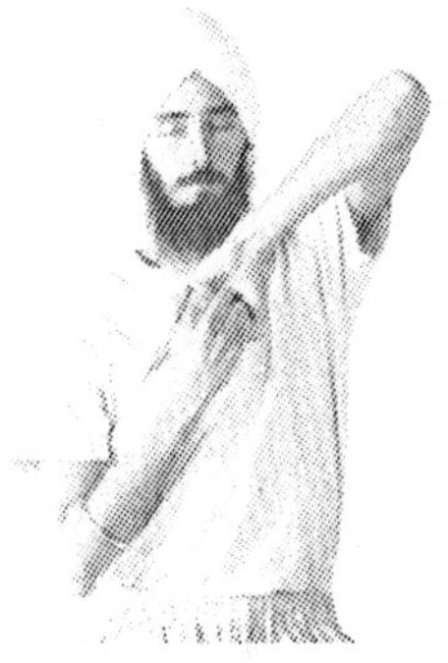

Hook the fingers of the right hand, palm facing in, over the curled fingers of the left hand (palm facing out). Moderately pull the hands apart in a bear grip while keeping the shoulders relaxed down. Inhale as the left elbow goes up and the right moves down, exhale as the arms twirl the opposite direction. Continue in a rapid movement. The hands stay relatively still in front of the heart center. Feel the arms as a propeller, opening up the heart. This is very rejuvenating. When finished, inhale, pull the hands apart and apply a Mhula Bhand, exhale, inhale and repeat keeping the shoulders relaxed and the neck straight.

8) Upper Spine Camel Ride : 1 to 3 Minutes

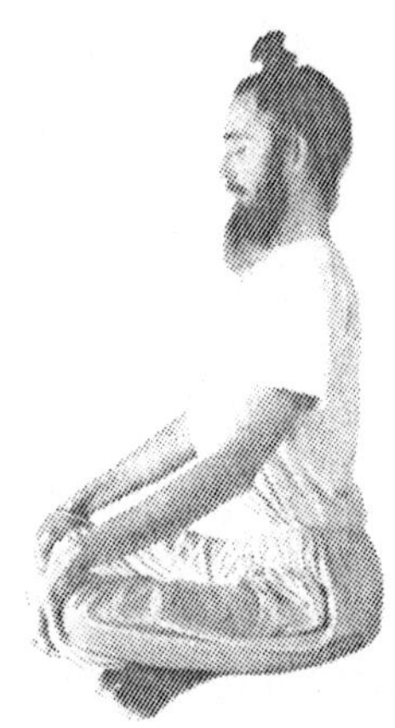

Sit in easy pose; hands on knees and arms straight. Flex the upper spine forward as you inhale, flex the spine back as you exhale. Head stays still. When finished hold the breath and apply Mhula Bhand.

9) Flapping arms : 1 to 3 Minutes

Arms straight to each side, palms down. Inhale the arms one foot up, exhale the arms one foot below horizontal. Move in a continuous spirited rhythm with a deep breath. Fly....

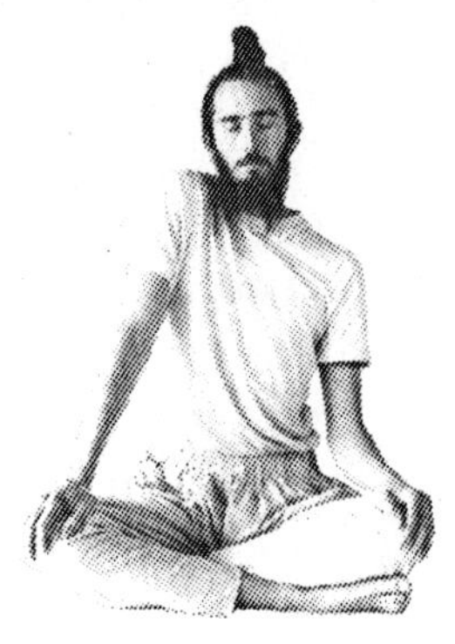

10) Shoulder shrugs : 1 to 2 minutes :

Inhale alternate shoulders up to the ears, exhale down.

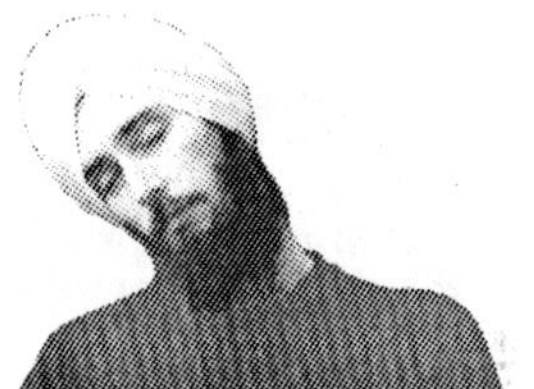

11) Neck Rolls : 3 to 5 times each direction

Let the head and neck totally relax as the head rolls around on its own weight. Inhaling as the head travels back, exhaling as it moves forward.

12) Over the Head Bear Grip, pulling

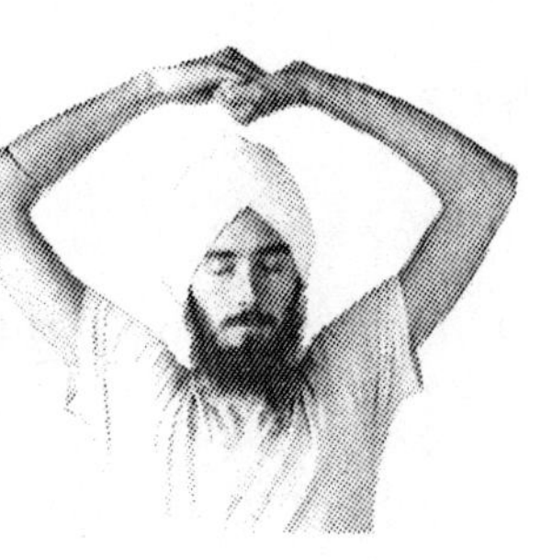

Sit on the heels and bring the hands six inches above the head in a bear grip, left palm facing down. Inhale deep and pull the hands apart while holding the breath and applying a Mhul Bhand for 15 to 20 seconds, bringing your energy up the spine. Exhale, hold the breath out while pulling the hands apart and applying a Maha Bhand. Repeat this cycle three times.

13) Sat Kriya : 3 to 11 minutes as described on following page.

14) Meditate : 3 to 11 Minutes **:** Calm, deep, and aware._**Move your presence and subtle breath up and down the spine.**

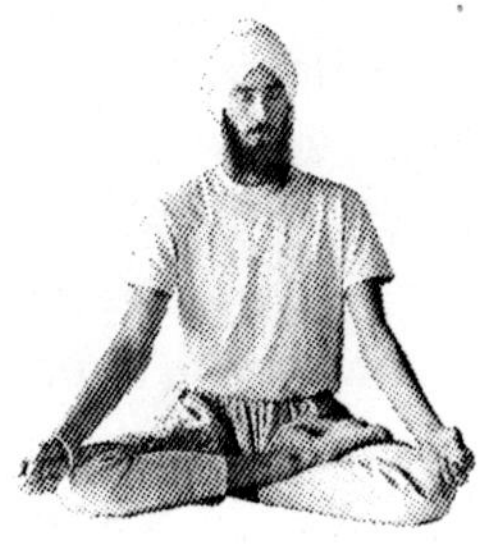

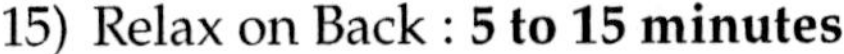

15) Relax on Back : **5 to 15 minutes**

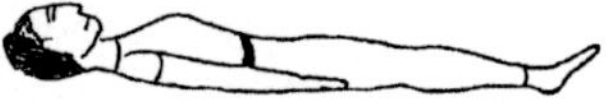

Sat Kriya

Sat Kriya strengthens vital energy and directs it upwards for the benefit of the entire body. The digestive fire becomes healthy, nerves become steady, and thoughts are clear.

Continual practise creates a sweetness in the body by refining the sexual juices into *Ojas*, an important oil necessary for the health of the brain, nerves, and spiritual grounding within the body.

Through rhythmic coordination of muscular contraction and relaxation, dynamic visualization, vibratory sound, and willful coercion, Sat Kriya magnetizes the spine and third eye as a seductive force to elevate the sexual energy of body and mind into spiritual awareness.

Sit on the heels and keep the spine straight. Bring the arms straight overhead, palms flat together. Do not get sloppy with the posture. If this is too difficult or if you are just beginning this type of Yoga, then interlace the fingers together into a fist and point the index fingers straight up.

Chant - **Sat Naam*** with much power from the navel. Sound a short **"Sat"** as you pull the navel in towards the spine and slightly up. The perineum and genitals are slightly contracted as well. It is important that the sound is made from the guts. The shoulders will move up a bit as the navel is drawn in to make the sound. Connect the energy from the navel all the way back to the spine.

* *Pronunciation:* The "A" in "SAT" sounds like the "a" in "father"
The "AA" in "NAAM" sounds like the "a" in "vietnaam."

Chant **"Naam,"** while relaxing the muscles and directing energy up the spine into the head. You may want to let some energy continue up above the head and rain back down into the body.

Continue at a rhythm of about 20 repetitions per minute. A slight breath sneaks in before the sounding of "Sat."

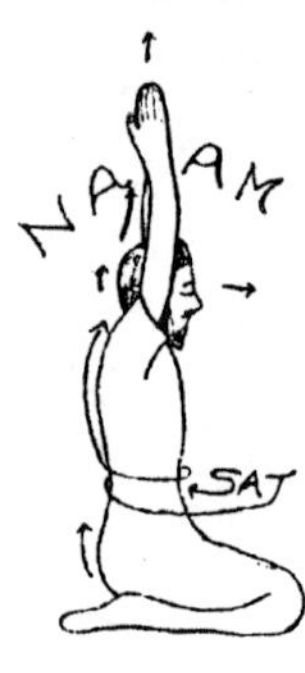

When finished, inhale deeply, keep the arms stretched up and hold the breath as long as comfortable while applying a **strong** *Mhul Bhand* and *Neck Lock*. Exhale, Inhale and repeat. Inhale, exhale and hold breath out applying a full *Maha Bhand*. Inhale, stretch the hands briefly overhead, and then meditate for a few minutes, keeping awareness of the spine. Travel easily up and down the spine with your mind. If you feel a contraction anywhere, then bring a sensation of ease and openness to that area.

Allow yourself to integrate the energy you have created. Do not drink liquids, or take a shower for at least 15 minutes and move in a contained fashion.

As a daily practice start with 5 to 11 minutes. After one week add 1 minute every one to three days. Build the time slowly.

This Kriya generates a heat that makes its easier to feel and thus keep your attention on the movement of energy up the spine. Internalize this heat, bringing it into the marrow of the spine (several inches under the skin). Sensing the spine opposite the navel helps to internalize energy and ignites the feeling itself. Experiment with different places within the spine, such as about four inches below the navel. As you do this it will possess both a warmth and a refreshing cool quality. If you do not feel this at first, just imagine it. As long as you remain one-pointed and focused then you will contain and direct your energy, and in time you should definitely feel a very tangible effect.

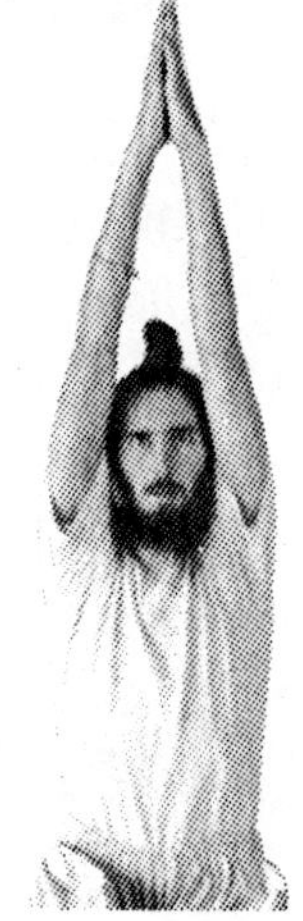

While doing this practice it is advisable eat a simple diet including greens and cooked whole grains. It is advisable for a man to contain his seed during this practice and for a woman to circulate and feel her own energy. This is definitely not a practice for women on their moon cycles or while pregnant.

Variations of Sat Kriya

1) Sit in full lotus or in celibate pose (between the heels).

2) Lie on back, legs crossed, arms straight above chest, palms flat together.

3) Sitting cross legged, lower the forehead to the floor and raise the arms as high as possible behind the back. Either interlace the fingers together into a fist or place palms flat together. Do not apply the breath at the end in this variation.

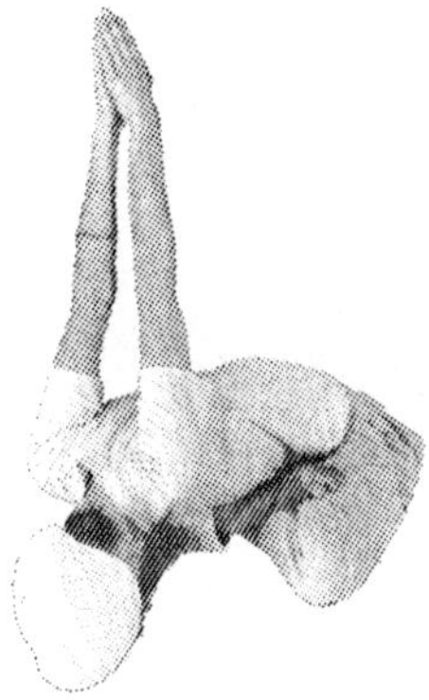

4) Sit on the heals in a bath of warm water up to the navel. This helps to further detoxify the body.

Rejuvination is Youth

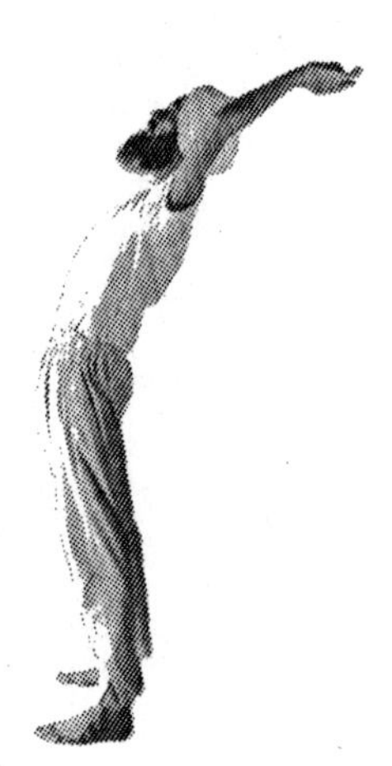

1) Backwards Bend : 3 minutes

Stand up, stretching the hands over head. Curl the little fingers against the palms and hold them down with the thumbs. Lean back, eyes open. Create a stretch across the chest. If you get dizzy stop. Helps to rejuvenate blood and stimulate the thymus.

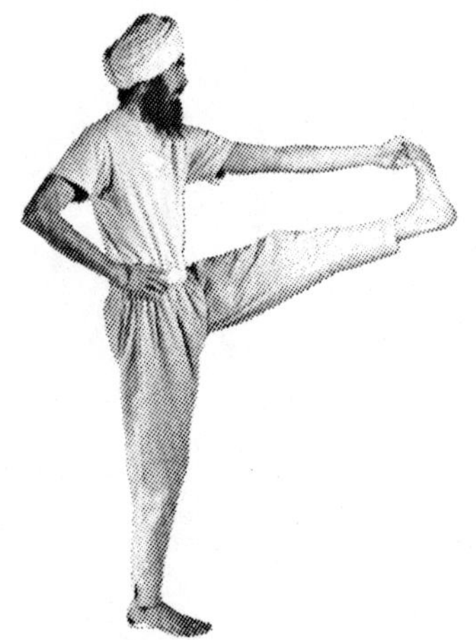

2) Stand on right leg and hold left leg straight in front with hands holding on to the foot, strong deep breathing. 4 minutes, then repeat on other leg. Good for potency and ability to follow through with conviction.

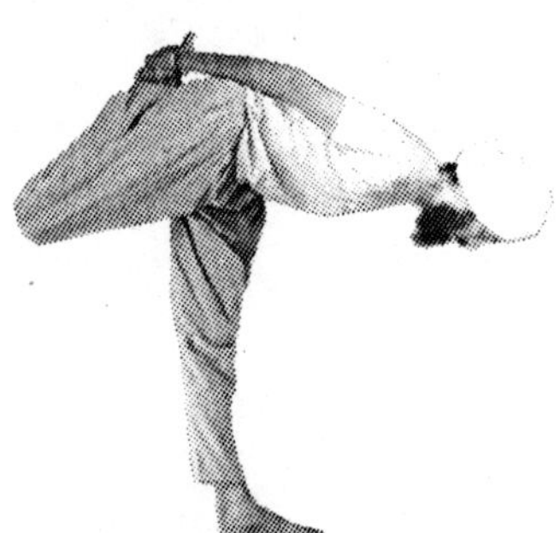

3) Bobbing : 2 minutes

Stand on left leg and hold your right foot against the buttock. Left hand holds onto the right elbow. Keep the spine straight as you bend forward to horizontal and back up again.

4) **Stand with legs spread wide apart.** Twist the body and touch the right foot with the left hand. The other arm is straight up overhead, in line with the right arm. Great for the liver. 2 minutes.

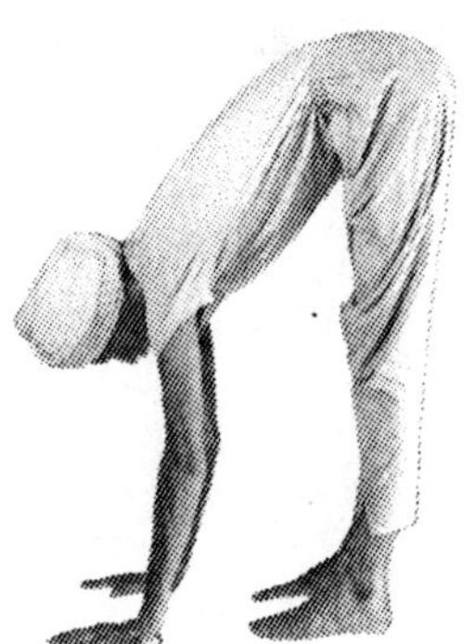

5) **Standing,** place heels together and angle feet 60 degrees. Bend down with straight legs and place hands flat against the floor. Inhale through the mouth, exhale through the nose. Equal weight on the hands and feet. 5 minutes with a strong breath.

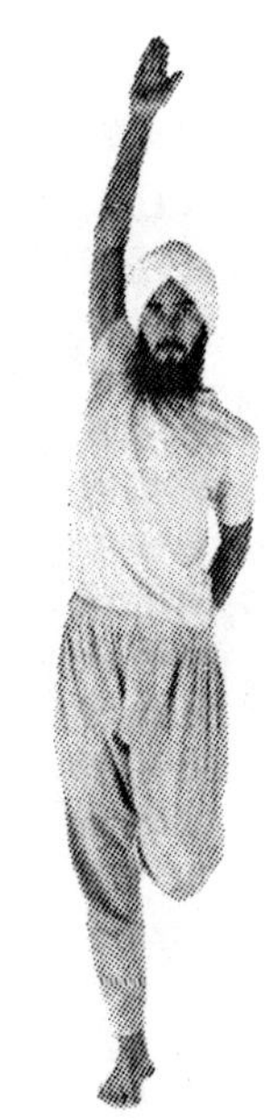

6) **Stand on the right leg** and hold the left foot against the buttock. The right arm is straight overhead, palm facing forward. Keep the body straight. Open the mouth wide and do a strong Breath of Fire. Move the navel dramatically and with force. 3 minutes.

7) Bowing : 11 to 31 minutes

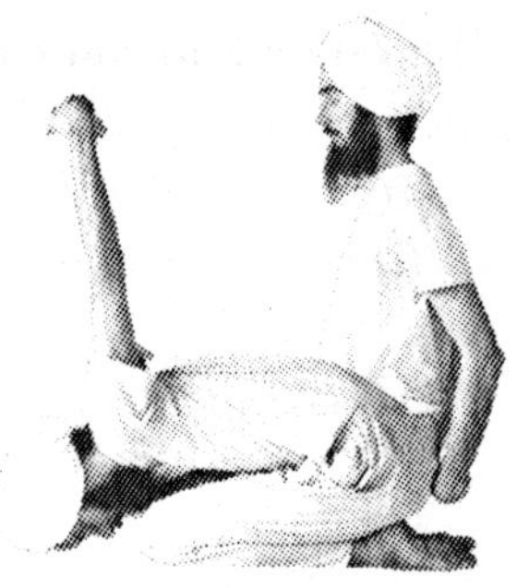

Sit on the heels, hands interlaced into fist at the small of the back. Inhale as you lower the forehead and raise the arms up, exhale to original position. Move at a quick tempo of the following 10 count rhythm. Inhale down and exhale up 4 times for a total of 8 counts, then remain up for 2 counts feeling your composure with a straight spine.

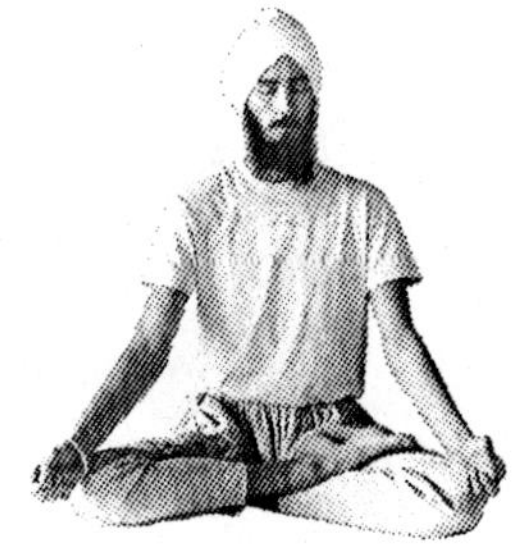

8) Meditate : 3 to 5 minutes

9) Sitting with a straight spine straight and extend both arms straight out in front, palms facing down. Move the right arm up 90 degrees and back down to horizontal. Move fast, and as you warm up, move faster, and faster. Excel by constantly applying yourself. The other arm and the rest of the body stays absolutely still. In that stillness observe the activity of the right arm, and move it fast. 5 minutes.

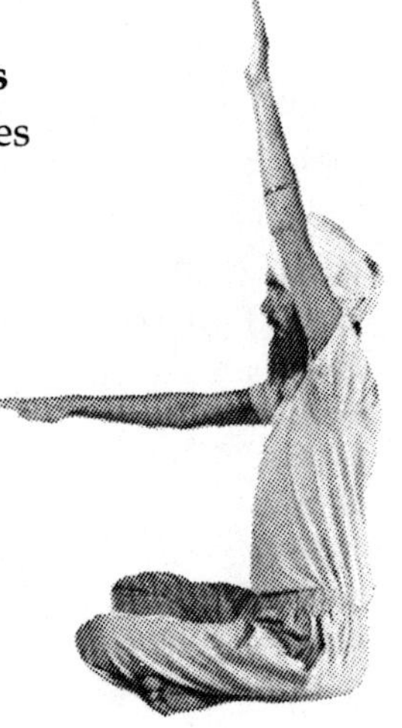

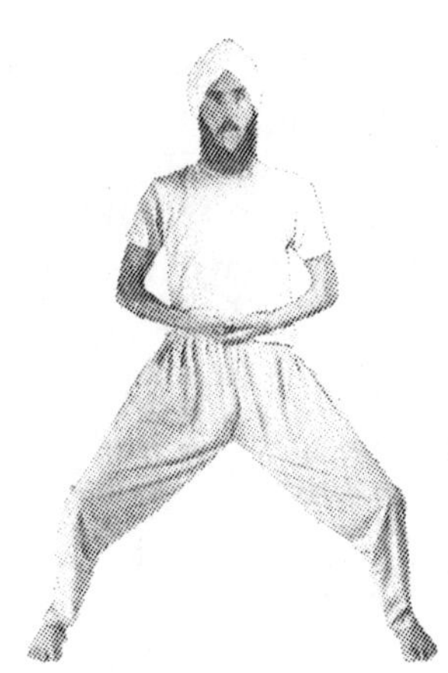

10) Stand up and come into a horse stance by placing feet about two feet apart. Bend the knees, as if you were sitting on a high chair. Cup the hands together in front of the navel, the sides of the hands touching just below the navel. Open your mouth and start moving your tongue in and out rapidly. Keep moving it quickly. 2 minutes.

11) Relax on back : 15 minutes

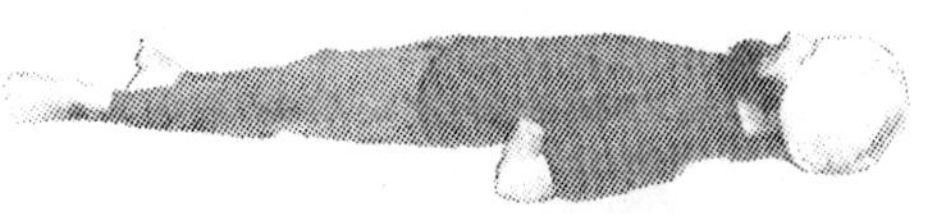

Here is the secret: place the hands with palms against the floor underneath the small of the back. Move into a total relaxation.

12) Rapidly Crossing Hands : 3 to 8 minutes

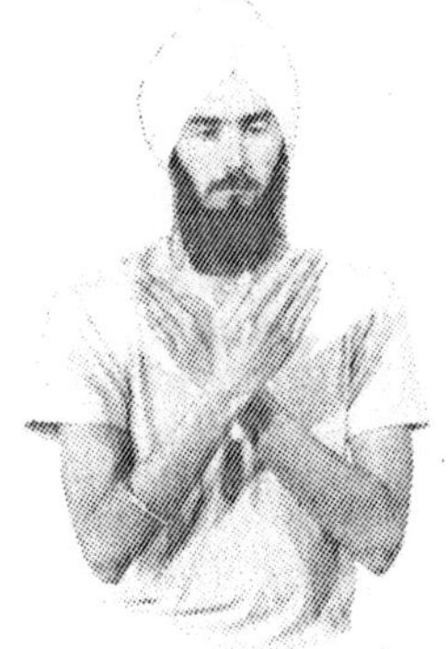

Sit in easy pose. Bring the hands in front of the face, palms facing in. Keep the hands very flat and stiff. Moving from the elbows, begin crisscrossing the hands, alternating one in front of the other, keep going, moving faster than you think you can. When you are at top speed, then surrender and move faster. Every time the hands cross imagine that you are creating flowers. Sit in a mountain of flowers, raining flowers, creating beauty and clarity every time the hands cross.

13) Waving Good-bye to the past : 2 minutes

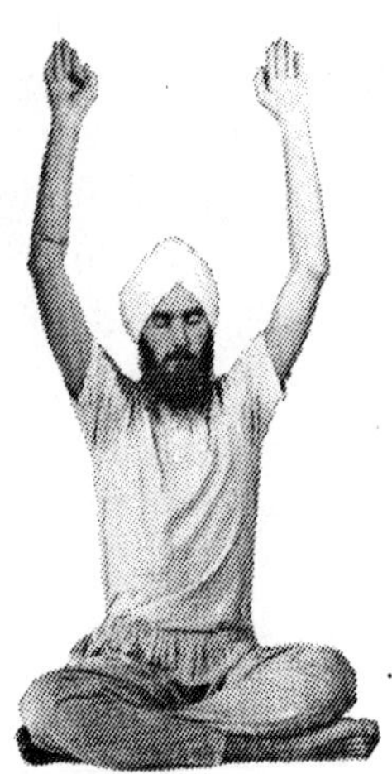

Sit up, put your hands straight up over your head, and wave them. Wave good-bye to your past, to problems imagined in limited consciousness. Wave good-bye to past images of relatives and friends who have died. Wave good-bye to your problems, fears, and ambitions, and wave hello from your heart in a new light of your rejuvenated self which supports your expanded awareness of universal reality. **Feel happy.**

14) Future Projection of Perfection : 5 minutes

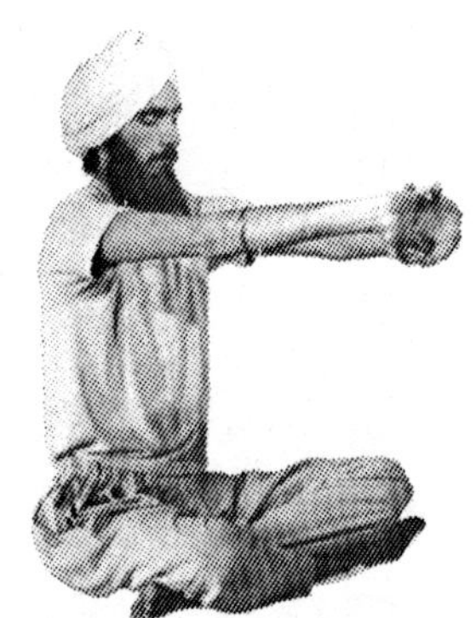

Interlace the fingers, and extend your arms straight out in front, palms facing out. Close your eyes, sit straight. Bend forward a few millimeters, and not more than that. Develop the feelings that you are still moving forward, and launch yourself, imagining that you are flying through time and space. Hold the feeling of moving forward, and the expansion. Feel you beauty, your freedom, your truth. After five minutes, inhale, hold the breath to capacity, and continue to project with the thought that ***"I Am Perfect, I Am Beautiful, I Am a Beautiful Being ..."*** Feel your projection and its creation.

15) Rolling on Back : 1 minute

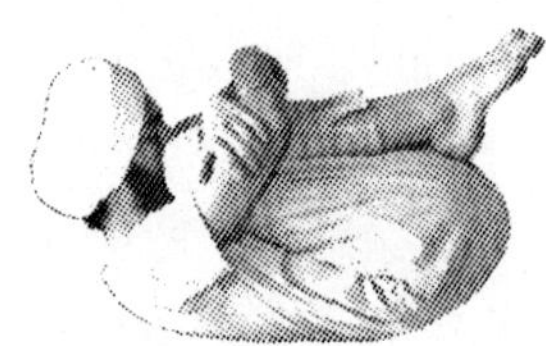

Lie on the back, hold the knees against the chest and roll on the spine, back and forth. Roar as a lion!

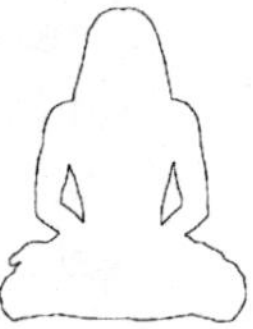

10

Martial Stances and Chi Kung

This chapter presents Martial Art Stances as a spiritual practice and Chi Kung exercises

Martial Arts Stances

A stance is a way of standing that gives a stable footing on the earth, enhances our energy and communicates deeply with our environment. A stance has at its root stillness around which movement may revolve. Employing a stance within our practice builds a foundation in which to expand and taking a stand (or a stance) gives us the definition in which to be awake and thus evolve.

Martial art stances can be used as a standing meditation that roots spirit into your body and your body upon the earth. Chi Gung is a Taoist practice of energy cultivation often using posture, breathing, hand movement and visualization, although there are some forms of chi-kung that use only the mind through internal pathways of cultivation.

Practicing chi kung in a martial stance is a very effective way to:

- Fill out your life force in both quality and quantity. In the process you will clear blockages and balance the emotions.
- Strengthen the body and center yourself in your vital centers. Gets you out of your mind and into your body through a union of mind and body. Improves your relation to the earth.
- Of particular value is how stance work teaches you about (and helps to correct) symmetry, such as the symmetry of the two sides of your body, of the front and back, of up and down. Symmetry, through balance, opens the gateways into refined consciousness. Symmetry will align your posture. The benefit of improving symmetrical awareness has vast and great benefits in our spiritual practice.
- Move beyond the dualities of pain and pleasure in the body to experience the stillness within all movement. Cultivating awareness of spirit in matter.

The first step is to gain competence with a stance in which to base your practice. It is best to start standing perfectly still in a stance (rather than moving the arms, etc.), because your attention will be more directed to mastering the stance itself, which must be correct before the full benefit of the stance can be gained. Just standing in a stance is a tremendous benefit in itself, and by learning to sit into it teaches you a lot about your body and the emotions that shape it.

I strongly recommend getting assistance in learning the stances and having them checked regularly for correct alignment. Look for an instructor or experienced practitioner in the internal martial arts for this, even if you have no intention of practicing stances for their martial applications.

I have found that the practice of the stances go hand in hand with Dynamic Yoga. While this yoga is complete without the practice of the stances, they give an extra strength and grounding that is tremendously helpful. For those wanting to explore further in the martial arts, I believe it is more important to base your decision on a style according to the teachers available, i.e., you will get much more out of a good teacher perhaps in a style you would not have initially chosen, than an attractive style and a mediocre teacher.

Stances are basically standing positions of a solid footing upon the Earth. While there are many ways of standing, the principle stance for our purposes is the moderately wide horse stance whereby one stands with feet apart with bent knees and a straight spine. The farther apart ones legs, the more emphasis on muscular strength and the lower back as a source of power. The closer in the legs the more soft energy is used to hold the stance and a greater emphasis of drawing energy from the Earth. Stances with the legs touching down to the knees, and stances with the legs very wide apart are the most difficult (the extremes), however stances with the legs closer can be safely done for longer periods of time as soft energy is unlimited, thus when we know how to use this the joints are protected. I have seen a number of not overly athletic woman hold the Buddha-hand Wing Chun stance (with the knees touching) for a half hour much easier than athletic men with martial arts training, and the men are baffled at how they can do it so much easier than them, as this is a difficult position to hold. It is because women tend to understand how to surrender and how to use soft energy more than men. So understand that even though stance work may seem really tough it is not just brute force.

All the stances use the lower tan-tien, i.e., an area just below the navel as their center of gravity and grounding strength. In all the stances, energy from your kidneys comes into play. This is one if the reasons that stance work is so rejuvenating and healing. The feminine stances in particular need the additional opening of the frontal line and thymus to sit in them correctly for longer periods of time. When the feet are held slightly more than shoulder width apart, with feet pointing straight, a good balance of masculine and feminine strength is used in the stance.

Some martial style stances will turn the feet in, emphasizing the inside of the legs and the frontal line as a source of power and to protect the groin area. Some will turn the feet out, emphasizing a different line of power through the legs. Each is valid, particularly with further refinements of how to direct your energy received from an instructor. A good balance for our purposes is to point the feet straight.

Warm up before beginning with a few stretches and running in place. Start with the amount of time that you can hold the posture correctly without fidgeting such as looking down or bouncing. From the very beginning do not look down constantly or bounce up and down. If you really need to relieve some pressure form your knees, then move them in and out in a sideways direction a few times, or shake the legs a bit, purposely, but do not constantly fidget through your mind not being able to remain focused within your body. Your feet should contact the earth firmly, on all points, with a balance between the front and back.

Then slowly increase the length of time according to your ability to hold the stance correctly. At times you may ask a friend or use a mirror to check that your spine is straight, your hips are tucked in correctly and that you are evenly placed over the feet.

Grip the earth firmly with the feet and keep all parts of the foot firmly against the ground with even pressure, particularly a balance between the front and the back. Occasionally, while standing in a stance claw the earth with your feet, to get the feeling. Remember not do look down while doing this, just keep the eyes normal and looking forward. In terms of the eyes, it is best to keep them relaxed, soft, yet alert. With few exceptions never close your eyes. While closing the eyes is a good way to internalize our energy, in stance work we are creating a balance, a total integration. Trying to escape from discomfort in this case is not what we want to do, rather we want to go through it and out the other side. So to repeat, do not close your eyes as a way of escape. Besides your stance will likely become sloppy. If my teacher saw that our eyes were getting glassy or disconnected, he would simply give a little nudge on our legs and we would loose our footing. This was because in the process of trying to withdraw, the attention is not on the circulation of energy and the root is lost.

Keep the spine straight and "suspended" by sinking from base of the spine into the ground and at the same time feeling that you are being lifted up from the top of the head. Shoulders spread apart and relaxed down. Neck straight. Look straight with the eyes relaxed. The legs will burn, maintain you composure throughout by relaxing into it and using soft energy. Shaking of the legs and the hips is a very good tonic for the nerves and a purification of the body. Over time from the navel down will feel rooted and as strong as an ox, and the upper half of the body will feel light, infinitely responsive and full of energy.

For a person of average fitness, practice for several weeks for about five minutes every other day. As the muscles become toned, then sit longer in the stance and go through the shaking. Do not sit longer than you can correctly hold the posture. Add on a minute every other day, or even every week and build the time. Building to and then maintaining fifteen minutes is fine for most people. As a more intense practice build to 30 minutes or an hour, each day.

You may see advanced martial arts practitioners doing their standing forms in what appears to be a shallow stance. However these practitioners have cleared there blockages, achieved an integration, know how to root their energy deep and wide, and they have done years of deeper stance work to help develop this ability. Unless you have physiological problems such as a damaged knee that prevents it, it is better to practice deep. This also generates a lot of energy that can be directed and it teaches us how to move past initial pain into a union of mind and body (which has a bliss to it). Yet do not try to master a deep stance all at once. Never push a strained ligament or knee. Be consistent, not fanatical.

Sifu (See-Foo) is a title given as a respectful term to ones martial arts instructor when that being becomes a profound guide. Its literal translation is like a spiritual father. Khalid Kareem, who was my Sifu in the martial arts taught us that one must always start gradual so that what he calls the small or psychic muscles/ligaments can become toned and clear. Then these small muscles can help hold the bigger muscles in the correct alignment so that our energy and awareness moves through them appropriately. Otherwise if we push too quickly in the beginning, besides risking injury, our small muscles will collapse and the big ones will try to do it all on their own. This becomes a brute force approach that lacks the necessary alignment. The small muscles, fascia and ligaments do not primarily hold the big muscles in structural alignment through mechanical means, rather they also help connect the flow of energy through our bones, organs and inner spaces into outer manifestation through the large muscles. Thus the simple act of standing in a deep stance has much to teach us through inner awareness.

Muscle tone and alignment is one side of the coin. Another is building a reserve of soft energy in the body that is initially circulated through the small orbit (this is the microcosmic orbit which is given later in this book) and then through the legs and arms, and into the earth and environment. The chi-kung movements given here are aspects of improving circulation and building of energy. Often the term "cultivation" will be used. Cultivation is the building, refining and circulation of energy. As this is a book on cultivating the nectar body, it is filled with practices to build, refine and circulate energy into nectar substance.

Throughout the stance pull up and tighten the perineum and the anus. Sometimes tighten the buttocks as well. Feel vitality at the Tan-Tien, which is a point about two inches below the navel and one and a half inches inside. As you feel that you gain centering and substance from the Tan-Tien then move the tan-tien deeper into the body towards the spine. As you continue the stance feel a rich and full strength emanating from your lower back, which you can emphasize through Mhul-Bhand (pulling up the anus and perineum) and learning to breathe in through the kidneys. Strengthening and connecting with the kidneys is one of the prime benefits of stance work. When finished, slowly walk around and feel your connectivity to the Earth. Next stand for a few minutes centering in your lower abdomen and just feeling good. Then lift the knees alternately to the chest a dozen times to help eliminate soreness, perhaps dance for a few minutes.

There are two ways to breathe known as normal and reverse breathing. In both types of breathing we inhale our breath down into the lower abdomen thereby extracting energy more efficiently from the breath for use by the body and spirit. In normal breathing as we inhale the diaphragm drops down and the lower abdomen expands outward. As we exhale the diaphragm rises back up and the lower abdomen sinks in. The breath is not forced to be too big, just natural, easy and full. This is the normal, healthy type of breathing used in almost all the exercises and practices in this book

The second way is called reverse breathing or Taoist breathing. Basically as you inhale the diaphragm down, instead of expanding the lower abdomen out, you draw it in. At the same time the lower back expands out more so than it commonly does in normal breathing. This helps to fill the kidneys with energy and make the whole kidney area feel more open. As you exhale and the diaphragm rises the lower abdomen pushes out. This pushing out on the exhale can be used as to give extra force to energy moving through various routes, which is the main reason it is used. Simply reverse breathing is more effective at propelling energy. Remember to expand the kidney area as you exhale, otherwise you will feel that you are suffocating.

For marital purposes reverse breathing keeps the frontal line stronger and projects less of ones intentions to an opponent. As a variation for this purpose there is very little visible movement at all in the abdomen, rather there is an internally contained expansion in the lower abdomen that can be seen solely though the lower back expanding out. This is given for educational purposes and for our application we can ignore this.

Until blockages in the solar plexus are released and the lower back loosens up reverse breathing can seem tough and unnatural. Thus practice a little at a time, use stretching and various practices to loosen up and gradually gain the capacity. Also remember do not try to make the breath super big, just natural. It is not just the amount of oxygen we are getting from the breath that is important, rather the energy extracted from it. I have heard of Taoist and Tibetan practices whereby a person can run a kilometer on just a few breaths and can run long distances effortlessly without apparent muscular strain. Obviously there is more at work here than just external air. As it becomes second nature, you can move effortlessly between the two types of breath.

An esoteric aspect of reverse breathing, introduced here for informational purposes, is adding a very smooth feeling of inhaling the energy within a thin stream, as if sucking the energy up through a straw, which can be the spinal marrow and inwardly the central channel, or inhaling it in the same thin stream down into the gut. In fact a foundational kriya used within the kriya lineage of Mahavatar BabaJi and Lahiri Mahasaya, while not employing reverse breathing per say, is very similar to reverse breathing in how it directs the prana through the breath.

When coming out of a horse, wing chun, eagle or a similar stance, first bring the legs together keeping the knees bent. Inhale as you bring the hands by the hips, palms up. Then in a slow and very focused manner, exhale as you turn the hands over (facing the ground), and straighten the legs while simultaneously pushing the breath through the hands and legs into the ground. As you do this the arms will also straighten.

This covers the basics. There are many more fine points that you can learn from an instructor if you want to take these techniques further.

HORSE STANCE - normal width

This is the basic stance most widely used for chi kung. Stand, with the feet slightly more than shoulder width apart. You may measure the width by twisting to the side and kneeling down on one leg, so that the knee touching the other foot. This is the correct distance. Stand up, bend the knees and sink into the ground. Tuck the hips in so as to straighten the curve in the lower back and increase the power by applying Mhul Bhand. Feet and knees may be:

a) Angled very slightly outward or straightforward. Knees out, as if bow legged, which gives a feeling of the position being "locked." Imagine from the knees to the feet as two big screws that bolt into the ground.

b) Feet facing forward or very slightly angled inward. Knees are not swayed to either side.

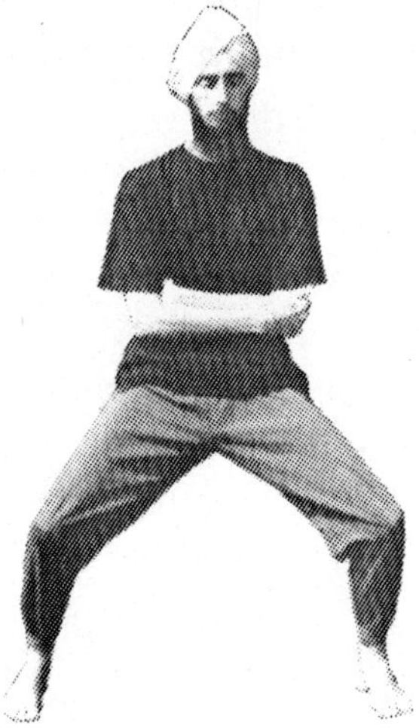

WIDE HORSE STANCE

Stand with the feet three feet or more apart, either facing straight out, or turned slightly to the outside. Bend the knees, and sink down. Keep the spine straight, hands resting on the hips. Look straight (not down). Breathe long and deep, or breath of fire. Stay steady (not bouncing up and down). Develops masculine strength. Practice for about 5 minutes (less if you are just starting).

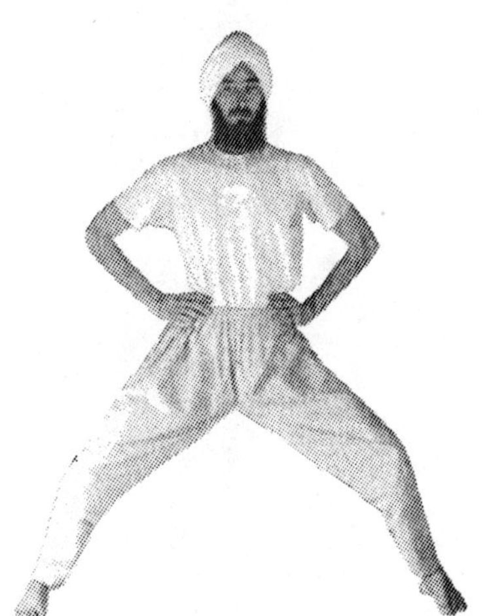

WING CHUN INVINCIBLE STANCE

This is the most internal of all the stances presented here, and one of the more difficult. Start with five to eleven minutes, then have the stance checked by a practitioner before increasing duration.

Stand straight, feet together. Bend at the knees. Keeping the heels together, angle the feet out, so that the big toes are the distance of the hand (fingers and thumbs stretched apart) width apart from thumb to tip of little finger. Then keep the toes where they are and move the heels apart, so they are two hand widths plus three finger widths apart. Stay sinking down, keeping even pressure on all parts of the feet touching the ground. Feel your feet are gripping the ground. Energy is drawn up through the bottom of the foot. Most important to keep hips tucked in.

Create a downward pull at the base of the spine by sitting into the stance, and at the same time an upward pull from the top of the head, so that the spine is stretched and suspended at the same time. Knees are bent in and touching each other. Press the knees together and sink them down. Look straight with eyes open. Arms are folded at the waist so that the right hand rest over the left side, and the right hand rest on the left elbow. Start with relaxed breathing, then do reverse breathing as described below. A tip: place a piece of paper between the knees and do not let go!

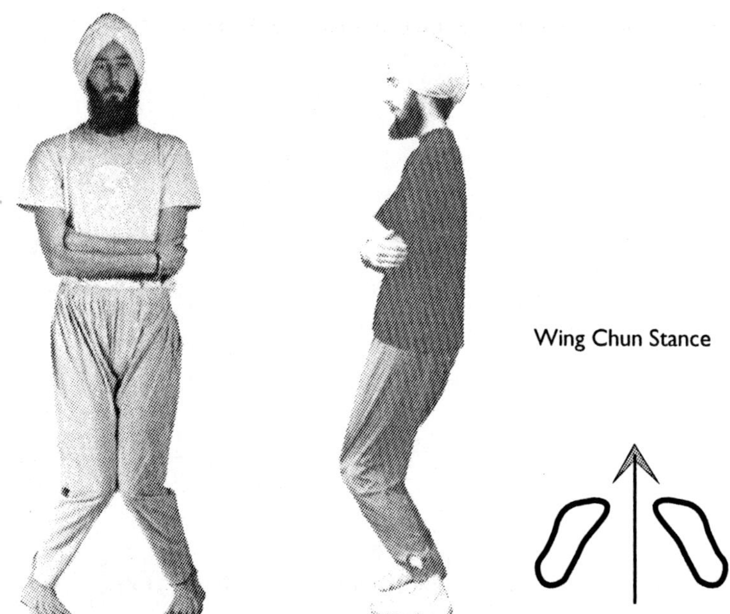

Wing Chun Stance

More on the Wing Chun Stance and mixing energy in the lower cauldron using the stance

Much of what is described here can be used as a chi-kung in the other stances, particularly the moderate width horse stance.

Wing Chun Stances the most feminine of the stances. For most people this stance is more difficult than a common horse stance both in the technique and because it uses muscles in a different way than most people are use to. It requires a deep grounding into the body. It does not require great muscular strength such as some of the super low stances, rather ability to work with soft energy. This stance is used in the martial arts to develop internal power for close in fighting, not just as pure strength but also to control ones own and the opponent's energy.

Each of the different styles of martial arts has within it different ways of practicing the style suited for its purpose, for example, scholar, merchant, military and religious forms. As I understand it, this form of the stance with the knees together is particularly used to develop a base within Buddha-hand Wing Chun, which is a seldom-taught style of Wing Chun that is used not just as a martial application, but as a moving meditation towards spiritual fullness. As such it employs an internal cultivation of energy, for which this stance is well suited.

According to my Sifu, Buddha-hand it is a rare fifth form of Wing Chun, beyond the religious form. To me, this says that there are truths locked within this lineage that transcends the confines of conventional scriptural application, i.e., this is a tantra and the domain of siddhas. These truths are not taught through books, or the forms of the practice itself, but through an inner touch and often through beings you may never meet in the physical.

In terms of all the forms, methods and martial applications, the stance is maybe one-percent of the content. But this is not a book on the martial arts, rather one that includes one of its foundational practices, this stance, presented within a spiritual perspective. Applied for this purpose and integrated with other spiritual practices, stance work has awesome benefit, far beyond just healing and strengthening.

Common transmission is the feeling and guidance gained during the course of practice whereby you "catch" the feeling, sensitivity and power of the particular practice. For example you watch how an adept does a practice. You are given little corrections. You do the practice over and over again and gain the feeling of it for yourself.

Profound transmission in regards to a practice is where the practice is just the conduit to greater understanding that transcends the practice itself. This is gained through the lineage of the practice and can occur in dreams, visions, very deep moments of clarity, and of course while practicing. This may be sparked through intensity, sincerity, joy, timing, the outpouring of our soul, and penetration.

Thus keep in mind that in doing this stance you are hooking up to a pattern that has been done by many masters before you. It is similar to how chanting a mantra that is dear to the heart of many masters connects you to them. You may want to gain instruction into the various forms (movements) done in the stance and in the moving forms of Wing Chun.

For example, in a number of very clear and profound dreams particular masters have shown me various tantras incorporating aspects of my practices. The forms were the conduits, but the essence was way beyond confinement to a particular form. It is not complicated, rather so simple, yet empowered. These forms are not just outer movements, but inner feelings and mixings, inner absorptions, bliss and the feeling of family. That is why you want to practice with full attention and pay a lot of attention to the details.

In the above use of the word tantra, I am indicating a continuum of our various forms of expression developed through the common core of the inner temple. I am also using tantra as an experience of the dissolution of outer perception into the elemental (fire, water, etc) display of consciousness that is the divine play of bliss as form characterized through the sambhogakaya body (the soul). I am using the word tantra in this particular experience as a kind of incredible blissful and awake dance.

In this way the eternal or ascended body is made manifest in consciousness, thus the term Buddha hand Wing Chun, or the continuum of buddhic consciousness into the physical body, i.e., the hand. Yet on a scholarly level, or martial level the term Buddha hand can have other meaning, such as the way the hand is held to direct energy through it, the power of the open hand in close in fighting and other meanings of which I am ignorant.

I am stating this so you may understand that there is a rich lineage behind these outwardly common and simply looking practices, and this lineage is inwardly available to those who practice with sincerity.

Stand with the feet about shoulder width apart and sink down. The knees touch and are held together. It is normally done with reverse breathing. Keep the hips tucked in so as to straighten the spine. Rotate the feet so that the toes angle inward. When standing without any arm movements, place the left hand over the liver area and the right hand over the left elbow. Sink into it and surrender. Sifu would sometimes place a piece of paper between our knees, and would say, this is your life, do not drop it. This is a great stance to practice the microcosmic orbit in. If you do not have someone to check your position that understands this stance, then it is better to practice the normal width horse stance.

I practiced it for a few years, first for a half hour, then for an hour each day with the standing wing chun forms along with general chi kung exercises and felt tremendous benefits from it. I do not claim to have developed it or the forms practiced in it to any degree of real martial perfection, but that was not my aim. While some people are naturally earthy, for myself I had to really work at it, to ground myself deep into my body. This stance gradually helped me to achieve this and showed me that very few people are perhaps more than 20 percent in their bodies. It also healed and straightened a curve I was born with in my spine. Clothes soaked in sweat, just holding it is tough, really tough, and then the energy drawn up from below and sunk from above mixes in the lower cauldron, the inner space starts to open and you feel so light, in bliss. The body may be shaking, it is still tough, but if you stay with it, it can become effortless at times. Your sweat starts to smell sweet. You may literally feel yourself disappear at times. Becoming so blissfully expansive and yet still be so grounded is hard to explain. Your perception of the world, the sense of ordinary struggle people live in, the sense that everything is solid and separate will never be quite the same. Even ordinary light looks different, more radiant, because your prana is cleaner and elevated and you are more open. This is a gift of this stance that you can take with you as experience. Experience is worth more than a million words. Taking this kind of experience into your meditation practices, such as eternal yoga and the higher tantras gives you the ability to advance much quicker. There is a Buddhist saying, "to hold the world in your palm."

As you get better at simply surrendering into and standing in the stance, learn to sink you energy into your lower abdomen, and draw your energy up into the same place. For myself it took awhile to learn how to really surrender and stand correctly, to obtain the right balance between inward absorption and outward attention. This is a wonderful benefit in itself and worth all the effort that goes into this practice even if no other benefits are obtained. So do not be in a hurry to advance before you get the basics.

To draw up, you have to sink down into the stance and through your perineum, legs and feet into the ground. To sink energy from above, you have to expand up through the top of the head. To remain stable you have to fill out energy horizontally around the navel region (the belt channel), which incorporates the strength of your navel. Through the intensity of shaking muscles and the necessity of surrender, you will create a nonverbal and exact cauldron in which the energy mixes. Stay with it. It is simple, nothing intellectual or complicated. After a month or two of getting the muscles fit for the stance, it may take five or ten minutes for the energy to reach this stage. There is no maybe, you will definitely feel it, so do not try too hard with your mind, just prepare yourself for it. If you are a man and do not learn to hold your seed, then it will take you much longer. The choice is yours; this is not about morality, just chemistry. Slightly push down the energy with the muscles of your upper abdomen and pull up with the muscles of the genitals, anus, and buttocks. At times inhale and hold the breath in this compression. At other times just breathe normally. Create a kind of potency in your tan-tien, but do not try too hard with your mind or make too much effort with your muscles. You build the energy, and then when it is ready, you squeeze it together and hold it in the cauldron of your lower abdomen. In some practice sessions you may hardly do this aspect of the practice at all, focusing instead on just being in the stance and perhaps doing moving arm exercises, in other sessions you will emphasize this mixing.

Then fan the fire-water-energy-substance, by staying with it. Keep it there, do not expand it too quickly; it will gradually expand out, up and down. If it goes away do not chase after it, simply return to the simplicity of presence. Let it develop over time and repeated practice. The first sign is the opening of an inner space deep in the body, not heat. Without that space there is no true cauldron, and there is no place for the energy to become enlightened, i.e., spiritual awareness. Remember that.

You do not have to generate the energy; it is already there from doing the stance. You simply learn to employ it in a skillful manner. The contrast of that light and easy space initially created through bringing energy together in the navel region with the effort of sustaining the stance is so great, that there is no mistake, and that effortlessness is a great incentive to find ways of converting the energy of the stance into inner vitality for this mixing and skillfully maintaining it.

Some readers might argue that this is not the true spiritual effortlessness, such as resting in the enlightened state, but we get there one step at a time, and I can argue back that such a reader has most likely not stabilized that experience themselves or they would not make that statement (true effortlessness has within it profound practicality of wisdom). It may stay with you as an after effect, like a tonic for much of the day. If in the stance, you loose the balance then you go out of your center and this makes things more difficult again which gives immediate feedback. As you will experience, stance work has a great system of built in check and balances. You learn through experience.

Learn to circulate the energy generated in that inner space into the microcosmic orbit. Your tailbone will likely make some big cracks when the energy moves through it accomplished by a greater sense of lightness. You may feel a kind of refreshing warmth move through tendons and joints deep in the body. This can be both a heat and coolness together and this is mystical. For example I will never forget the feeling when I first felt cool energy like a liquid heat move through the inside of my hip joint; like a first kiss. If you force energy out of the space in your cauldron too quickly, then the energy looses its mystical quality and becomes simply physical and in the process the inner cauldron disappears.

There is a lifetime of mastery awaiting us in the conversion of physicality into spiritual consciousness. Certain experiences perhaps sparked in this stance will be continued through other practices and life experiences in various modalities, refinements and times. For example, the initial mixings, the lightness and grounding, the experience of liquid light I tasted in the stance and kriyas took several years before other opening (pure buddhic awareness) occurred that brought everything together in a more meaningful way. Then another decade through other aspects of practice (greater definition and confidence through common maturity along with divine intimacy and transmission within the body of oneness) to come into a further state of fruition, and it will probably be more years for this to continue to its next stage, thus in this sense I am always a beginner.

All of this seeming greatness of experience itself dissolves in the simple radiance and joy of the oneness or emptiness. There is not much to talk about. In regards to the more impressive sounding details of your experiences, you may even forget that you have had them. This should tell you something of the beauty of where you are headed. Stating such experiences, besides being a helping hand, is simply to inspire you to practice, but the practices themselves, provided you do them, will keep you simple.

Likewise certain experiences sparked in other practices can be fortified into a greater stability through the stance. For woman do not practice the stance in your moon cycle and for a man learn to contain your seed, which will greatly add to your practice. This simple mixing of energy described for this stance can also be done in the horse stances.

In sitting or lying down practice our minds can get away from us, and there is no immediate physical penalty. But in a stance, when our mind gets away from us, it gets harder for we come out of our center. Of course you could always just stop doing the stance as a way of escape. So once you are fit enough, then when you make a commitment, stick to it. For example, say you are going to stand in the stance for 31 minutes. Then take a watch, and do not come out of it one minute early, no-matter-what. This will develop real grit and make your life easier in other ways. If you cannot stick to this, then do not make that commitment. Be honest but do not be afraid. Intensity can move us far on the spiritual path and give us real experience. The only exception is if you are aggravating a physical injury, such as a sharp pain, or you are suffering from an illness that you misjudged. For a woman, times right after her moon cycle can also be a reason to stop early. In these types of examples never be fanatical, for you are most likely only doing yourself harm. Another exception is in the case of true need of another individual, for example a parent with a small child.

You should not expect anything of grandeur; rather you have to work at it in the simple details; not letting the mind wander and staying present, naturally breathing, mixing, sensing, sinking, and just being present. In this way you cultivate the magic and it happens in its own time, but it may take much patience.

Of course in using a stance for spiritual development we also employ other means such as formal sitting meditation, dream transformation and awareness, kriya and a good nature. Think of the stance as like a motor or generator that makes a lot of vitality and cuts through excuses of the mind. You can use this vitality in all your other forms of practice, as well as empowerment for a good nature and joy of service.

Following are a few additional stances for strengthening and to open up energy.

EAGLES STANCE

Stand with feet and legs together. Bend at the knees, keeping the legs together. Place one foot about two or three inches in front of the other, keeping the sides of the feet touching. Look straight, hips tucked under, spine extended, shoulders apart and fold the arms across each other against the waist. This is a good training stance for the Wing Chun stance. Also sometimes when coming out of a horse stance, you first go into this stance for a minute, and then straighten up.

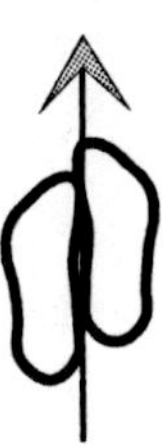

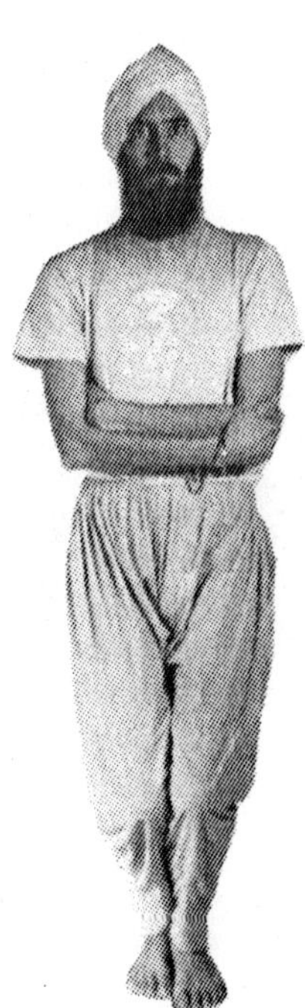

WARRIOR POSE

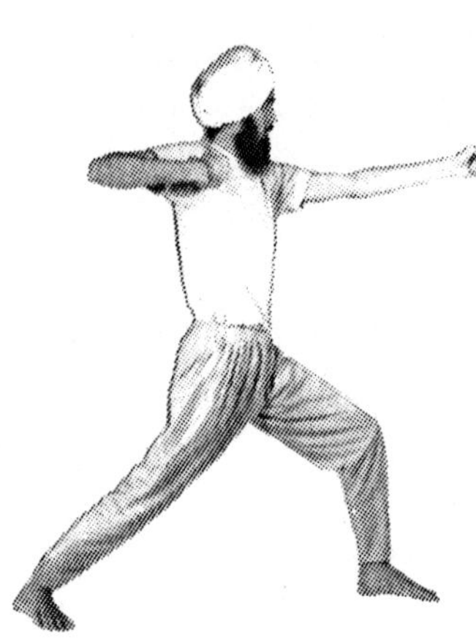

Stand sideways with feet apart as shown in diagram. Bend the front leg so that the knee is over the foot. The other leg is kept straight. Keep the spine straight and hips tucked in with the navel and torso facing forward. Hands either resting on the hips, or in archer pose, where one arm is extended holding an imaginary bow and the other hand is drawn back holding the arrow and string. Practice for a few minutes on each side for strengthening.

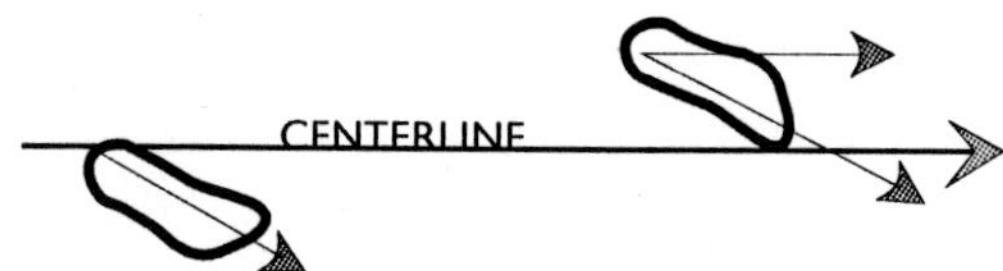

CHAIR POSE

Stand with feet just slightly more than shoulder width apart. Hold on to the inside of the ankles, so that the arms are on the inside of the legs, and bend at the knees so that the back is horizontal. Look forward, eyes and face relaxed. Increases potency and helps to open up the hips and genital area. Long deep breathing into the lower abdomen and groin, or Breath of Fire. Time: 2 to 5 minutes.

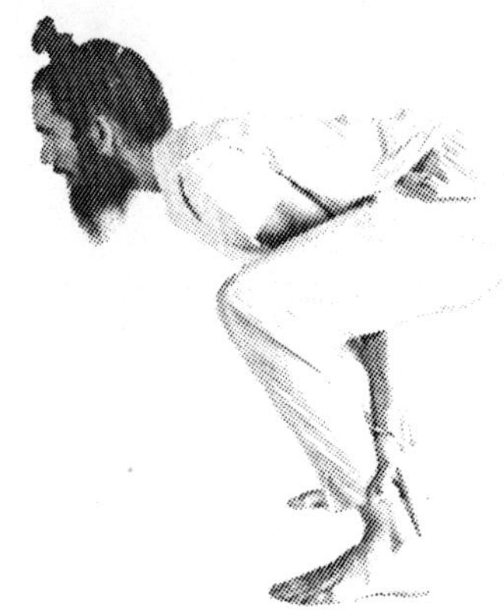

HORSE STANCE AGAINST A WALL

Helps with correct alignment of the spine and gives strength. Stand against a wall with feet apart in a wide horse stance. Heels are several inches out from the wall. Bend at the knees, keeping the back straight against the wall. Helps you in learning how to sit into a stance, which has the feeling of sitting down into a chair.

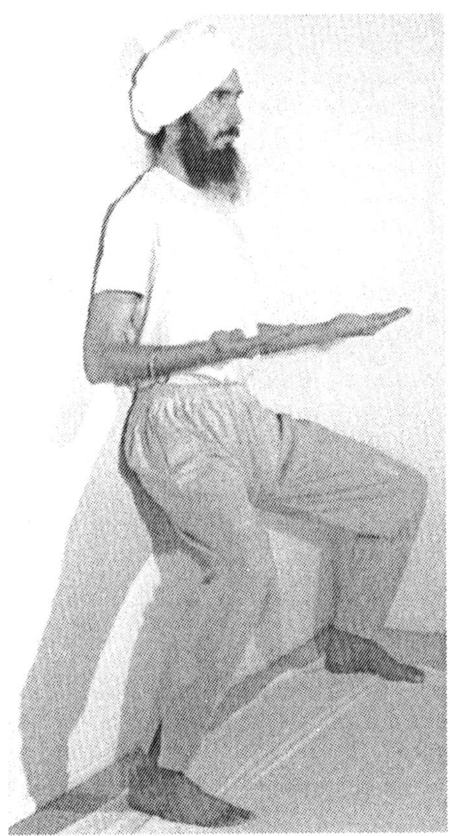

Chi Kung Exercises to do in Horse Stance

All of these Chi-Gung exercises are best done in a normal width Horse Stance. Keep all movements very slow and graceful.

HUGGING A TREE

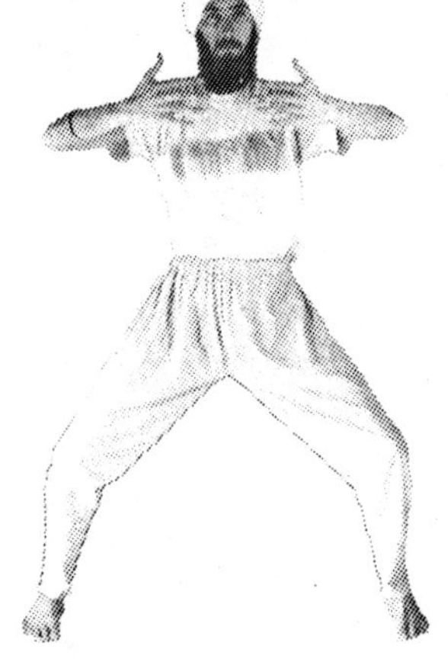

This could also be called, holding a ball. Practice the microcosmic orbit while holding the posture. Keep shoulders rounded, chest sunk in, elbows relaxed. The back is straight with a slight outward bow to it (rounding). Feel as if you are hugging a tree, with roots going into the ground. Look straight with relaxed eyes.

GATHERING CHI

Inhale palms facing up as the hands gather chi energy into the lower abdomen and up the torso as the hands move past the head. The hands gracefully turn outward as they move past the temples and then slowly exhale as the hands move down (palms facing down) to compete the cyclic motion. The hands move down about two feet out from the body so as to be ready to scoop up "Prana" into the belly as they turn upwards. Start the inhale as the hands begin to turn upwards as they again gather chi into the lower abdomen.

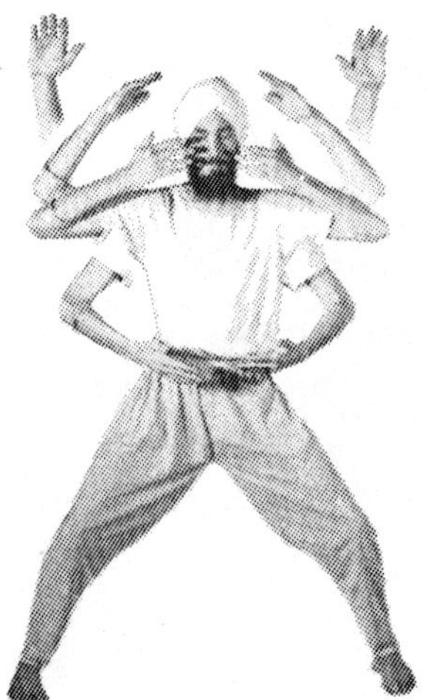

It is good to use reverse breathing with this chi kung. In you use reverse breathing, as you inhale, and the hands move up the torso feel that you are also inhaling the energy and breath up the marrow of the spine starting from the tailbone up into the head and to the third eye. Tighten the anus as you do this, particularly during the first part of the breath. As you exhale, bring the energy down the front.

POLISHING THE MIRRORS

This popular practice is very good for both opening the belt channel and also guiding prana from the torso into the arms and hands. Hands face down at waist level. Move the hands on a horizontal plane as if polishing two large mirrors. Keep movements slow and graceful. As the hands move towards the body inhale and feel a cool feeling on the inside of the arms. Exhale as they move to the sides and outwards feeling a warm sensation on the outside of the arms. Remember to keep the hands at waist level. This is good to do with reverse breathing, but if this is difficult for you, then normal breathing is fine.

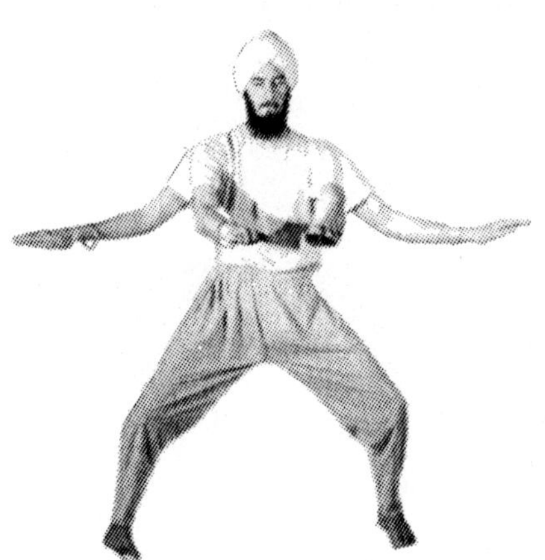

RUBBING ELBOWS

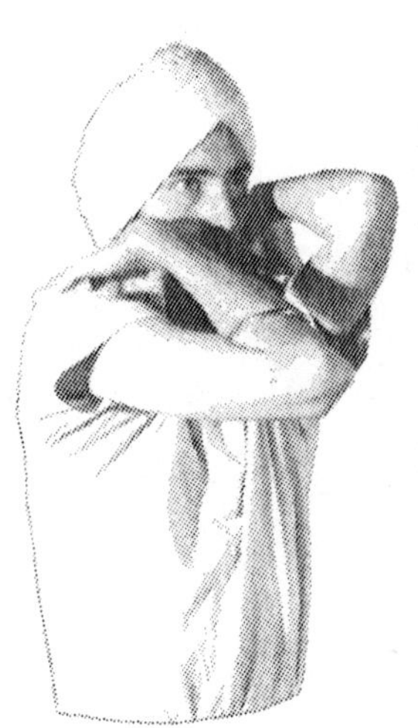

Hands on shoulders, move elbows in vertical circles, each elbow moving in opposite directions. As the elbows pass center they rub against each other. After going one direction for a few minutes, go the other direction. This helps to loosen up the shoulders and rib cage.

WAVING A HANDKERCHIEF

Movement and breathing is slow and graceful. Inhale the arms and hands to the position shown, as if waving a handkerchief. The head slowly turns to the side, eyes following the hands, being careful that the head itself does not look down. Just as the hands reach the position shown, flick the wrist so that the fingers point up, then exhale as the hands slowly move down to center. Inhale as they move up the other side, the head moving in coordination. This helps to open up the sides of the rib cage, which makes breathing easier and improves health.

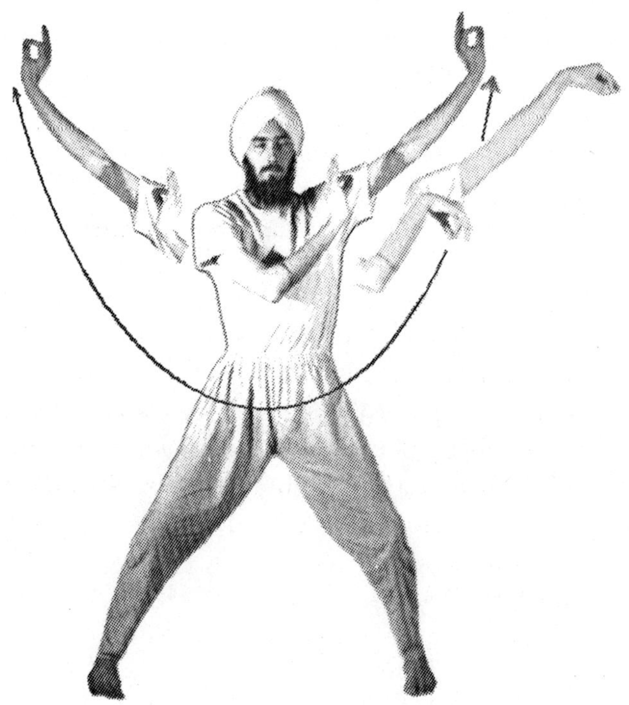

Gathering the Moon

This is a simple and enjoyable practice that is elevating, balancing, healing and grounding. Sometimes when you only have a few minutes, such as stepping outside for a stretch, or a few minutes before dinner, it is a good pick me up. You may like it so much as to practice it everyday.

There are many small moments in the day where we can practice exercises and/or mindfulness. For example, I like to stand in horse stance while brushing my teeth. Amongst countless additional examples; silently feeling yourself as a blessing presence while riding up in an elevator full of people; smiling; feeling the earth under your feet, noticing something; merging a mantra and awareness in common activities. Small moments like these add to the enjoyment and innocence of the day. They help to make your day more alive and they cultivates an atmosphere conducive to practice.

A dozen or two repetitions gives a nice effect, although do less or more according to your fitness, desire and acclimation to the exercise. Even stepping outside for 4 or 5 reps is beneficial. Keep the movements at a reasonably slow pace and graceful, connected one to the next. Pay particular attention to the movement of energy up and down the body. If you get dizzy, stop. Holding the breath for a short duration (a few seconds) is optional, but adds to the effect.

Do not hold the breath for a long time, particularly when arching over. Several decades ago in a related yogic exercise, in my enthusiasm, I would do exactly that while arching backwards. Thus one morning I found myself unconscious on the floor.

When you finish stand for a minute or two, and feel the effect. Gather your energy into the navel region. Then continue in your daily activities, ideally maintaining silence for at least a few moments.

1) Start by bending over so that your wrists are at about the level of your knees. Gently round your back. As you bend over inhale gently, then hold the breath for a short time and apply a light mhula bhand (tighten the anus and perineum). During the inhale and while shortly holding the breath feel your energy rising up through your feet and up through the spine, all the way into your head. Gently exhale while remaining bent over.

2) Then gently inhale as you slowly rise up, bringing your hands gracefully overhead (facing up) and arching backwards. The thumbs and index fingers of the hands outline a moon, which you look at. Hold the breath for a few seconds. During this upward movement the energy continues to rise up the body, and looking at the moon seems to enhance the effect, carrying the energy up and simultaneously softening it through the eyes.

3) Then exhale slowly through your mouth as you gently bring your body straight and lower the arms out to the sides. As the arms are lowered down, they are kept straight and point to each side of the body. While exhaling, feel your energy "gently" moving down the body to the ground.

4) Inhale and exhale once as you continue to feel energy flowing down from the top of your head through your arms and legs, and through the legs into the ground. There is no need to hold the breath for this part. While this is an optional addition, it gives extra time to feel the downward flow, which is an important aspect of this set.

5) Continue into the next repetition by inhaling as you bend over as outlined in step number one.

This particular chi kung exercise was popularized in an excellent book by Wong View Kit called "The Art of Chi Kung."

Massaging the Navel Area

While I have heard of this technique a few times over the years and upon reading a book on it by Dr. Yang Jwing-Ming I was inspired to practice it. This practice involves an initial building of energy at the solar plexus. After this area becomes very fit and full of energy the extra energy is led into the bone marrow. The biggest bone marrow in the body is the brain. Through continual increase and grounding of our energy into the bone marrow our strength increases and our perception becomes clear. This clarity combined with greater energy allows us to apply ourselves with great effect upon the spiritual path. For martial purposes legendary feats of strength and endurance can be accomplished.

After this initial cultivation of increase, transformation and circulation, there are further techniques to stimulate extra energy, such as massaging the genital area (not for erotic purposes), increased circulation into the large microcosmic orbit (essential for martial purposes), esoteric mixings of energy in the body and drawing in of cosmic forces. These will not be described here.

Dr. Yang's translates Bhodidharma's instructions of the full three year retreat for the practice along with notes and his wisdom. This includes three or four 90 minutes sessions a day. What is given here is a moderate version of the foundation practice, with some brief notes from my experience of it. Those who want to practice it in earnest should purchase the book *Muscle/Tendon Changing and Marrow/Brain Washing Chi Kung* by Dr. Yang Jwing-Ming and perhaps seek out instruction. Yang's book goes into this technique in much greater detail and gives a historical background. It also emphasizes the level of commitment necessary to successfully do this practice for those desiring the full effect.

I was doing this practice not for the martial benefits, but primarily for a spiritual benefit with a side interest in increased health to my navel area and thus geared the practice with my aims in mind and in relation to other forms of practice I was engaged in. While I only practiced it for eight months, each day consisting of two to three hours, and thus accordingly not to the degree subscribed in the book, I still found it extremely beneficial and could relate to the different stages talked about. I did not use the particular training methods described in the book for taking the energy into the large circulation (through the arms and legs).

Those wanting to do the full three year, 3 or 4 sessions per day practice as outlined in Bhodidharma's methods should seek out someone who has accomplished this for more complete guidance (not me, as I only did an abbreviation of it as described above.)

It has been said that massaging the navel region can heal many diseases and restore your organs to greater health. Immediate benefits include feeling good, a strong digestive fire, increased focus, and a profound sense of grounding.

These techniques are part of a larger system of energy refinement and control which have been practiced within the Chinese yogic arts for many centuries, similar to the way that kriya techniques are used to create clarity, vitality and grounding for use in either a greater goal of enlightened embodiment or for general well being.

Since energy and the mind are like two sides of a coin, one always leading the other, it is a common practice to use visualization to guide energy into our center and to refine it by the quality of our mind. Yet many of us are too scattered or too dull to be able to direct our mind for any length of time, and to accurately penetrate and radiantly hold it within the correct places or energy flows in our body long enough to experience real energetic transformation.

Some disciplines address this by emphasizing one particular area of the body to start with, such as the navel or third eye. After building, penetrating and refining the energy-awareness within this area, we can then spread it into our entire being. This is not a beginning or end step, rather a middle step. First we do general whole being practices, such as general exercise, basic meditation, purification and inspirational practices. Then we may focus intently on a middle approach, and upon gaining greater mastery use this strength to open up the rest of our being. By cultivating vital, incredibly alive energy, this takes us to a new level of radiant mind and teaches us the proper way of using our mind instead of our mentality.

In this particular technique we learn how to build up and refine energy in the solar plexus area. This includes teaching our body how to be a temple. For example, soft limitless energy requires soft, open, clean and energetically strong tissues to embody this energy.

Through massaging the navel area every day with hands and sticks, as will be described, your muscles and fascia become saturated with energy. At first this energy will be regular energy, but through working with it we transform it into soft energy. This soft energy can be better directed by our minds to where it is needed and stored in the body in large quantity. Soft energy is not just physical, but a quality of our being that is energetic.

The increased presence in your muscles and fascia gives you a reference that helps to firm and hold a focus deeper within the body. It becomes easy to maintain this focus without your attention spacing elsewhere. You can learn to direct this abundance of energy to clear blockages and as a means to greater awakening. In short, your feelings, mind, and potential all become profoundly connected. Start today by simply lying on your back with a pillow under your head. If it is cold, make sure to cover yourself. For women on their moon cycle, only do light to moderate massage.

Consistency is important. For those who want to approach this practice more casually, then start with ten minutes a day and gradually increase the time up to a half-hour. With this approach it is ok to miss a day here and there. Start with stage one and gradually incorporate all of the first three stages in each session.

If you want to radically increase the amount of energy that can be very tangibly directed through the body, then you must decide to practice once or preferably twice everyday for a minimum of six months using all the steps in each session. The exception is for women during their moon cycle. Of course a pregnant woman should not do this at all. With this approach, practice times will soon increase to between 60 to 90 minutes per session. It is vital that if you get into the more complete system you continue everyday without exception, because you will cause some of the muscles to become tight and a little swollen. The energy must move through this stage until the muscles again become soft, indicating that you have softened the energy being stored there and that you are able to absorb the energy into its center. If you stop half way through, the muscles can degenerate to a lesser condition than when you started. Most importantly you will not have achieved the potential of the practice.

Step One

I like to do a few warm up exercises first, although this is not critical. You should initially concentrate on an area the size of your hand between the navel and solar plexus. Begin with long strokes using the heel of the hand, moving from the right to left side (the direction of your intestines). This loosens up blockages and warms everything up. Then use a combination of back and forth movements with the palm of your hand and circular movements with the fingertips. Do not massage directly on the bellybutton itself.

Keep your attention focused in the area you are working, directly under your hands. Breathe easily into the muscles and tissues that are being massaged and while doing so feel or sense energy filling the area being massaged. Cultivating this directing of attention is very important, and in the long run the entire difference between being ineffective or effective in what you are doing. If your mind wanders, bring it back. This is increasingly important in the later stages of practice and develops soft limitless energy and awareness.

Develop perception of a soft containment of energy under the solar plexus area (several inches or more under the skin) that nourishes the whole area. Similar balls of energy may be felt under the navel and below the navel. Attune with the solar plexus energy as a white or golden-white sweet earthy quality.

Start easily at first and gradually increase the pressure and duration. Massage once or twice every day, and try your best not to miss a day. A person who is tight or sore in the stomach area may start with five or ten minutes. Otherwise a longer time is better.

After a week or more extend the area being massaged to include the area below the navel and under the lower ribs. Press down against the solar plexus with moderate pressure and breathe against that pressure. Be sure to feel that you are mentally energizing that area as you do the massage. As you progress, develop the feeling of an internal pressure in the muscles that pushes back against outer pressure. At the same time this energy is soft and pliable.

Step Two

The next stage of practice is after finishing massage, to slap the skin with your hands. Start just between the navel and solar plexus, extending to all the areas you have massaged. Over the weeks you can slap harder, yet it should never hurt (except a minor temporary sting).

When finished, smooth out the energy with gently massage and stroking. Slapping your skin greatly improves its resilience and your defense against external stress and sickness. However, it also drives quite a bit of energy outwards. As the principle aim after increase, is to internalize your energy, not drive it out through the skin, smoothing and relaxation should follow. When finished, cover yourself and relax on the back for a few minutes.

As you include the next stages, move the slapping, smoothing, and relaxation to the end of your routine.

Step Three

Extend the massage over the ribs. Work in-between the ribs with a finger(s) or a knuckle. Work from the solar plexus out to the sides. Massage up and down the sternum with a circular motion of your palm. Do the sides of the ribs thoroughly. It is a wonderful feeling when, through regular practice, the ribs do not contain any "charge." This improves your immunity. Be sure to slap this area as well.

Next turn on to each side and massage your kidney area, also slapping it when finished. !!! Start gently and progress gradually !!!

However, keep the main focus of energy and concentration in the solar plexus area. It is vitally important to understand that the feeling-visualization of the energy is the most essential aspect of the practice. It is the building up of this soft energy, at first barely tangible into a profound powerhouse that this practice is about. It would be of greater benefit to simply lie on your back and meditate on the energy, with no massage, than to let your mind wander while you massage and stimulate the solar plexus.

Decision Time

After doing the above for a month or longer, this is a good place to decide if you want to include the remaining steps of the practice. If not, then continue at your present pace until everywhere you massage is free of pain and feels really good. Once achieved, maintain it through practicing a few moments here and there, such as rubbing your stomach and chest area for a few minutes after awakening and keeping a good sense of vitality.

The above provides good health benefits without having to do the later stages. If you decide to go for it, the intensity will harden the muscles, even making them a little swollen. You must be very consistent until the muscles again become soft and you have integrated the extra energy smoothly throughout your body. Otherwise, if you quit halfway through, the muscles will most likely degenerate to a lesser state than when you started, and the opportunity will have been lost. The purpose of such intensity is to develop lots of soft energy, which you can then use for internal development and spiritual definition. As your energy moves into this quality, you will have both external and internal vitality, and thus a more balanced opportunity to forge forth into the higher tantras.

Moving to a greater level of intensity will gradually increase the amount of energy. This is to be absorbed into your body in a number of ways. The purpose of this practice is to guide the energy into your bone marrow so as to wash, energize, and enliven it with nectar qualities thereby allowing a great degree of both strength and spiritual awareness to become part of the body. For this particular practice the energy is drawn from the solar plexus outwards, i.e., the ribs, spine, etc. It is also absorbed through various channels, such as the microcosmic orbit and central channels. I also brought the energy into the tan-tien, and then into the navel chakra. If you do not understand how to do this type of absorption and circulation, then do not even think of doing this practice yet. Instead practice kriyas and do the microcosmic orbit to gain this ability. Everything in its right time, one to the next, will bring much better results. In the book it advises to be very careful not to lead the increased energy into the arms and legs prematurely during the first year (through practices such as various fist and intensive arm exercises), otherwise the energy takes on an outer show and this makes it difficult to fully awaken the inner structure. In my practice I did lead the energy through the legs as a container of excess energy at times (because I was directed in dreams to do so), but did not feel that this handicapped my practice in anyway.

Step Four

Get a metal ball such as the hollow balls used for Chinese hand exercises. While doing the massage place the ball under you buttocks to warm it. While a rubber handball is useful, I find that scent of the rubber disagreeable.

Roll the ball between your hand and the skin. Start with light movements and over time gradually go deeper. Also massage the ribs and between the ribs. Massage the solar plexus area, being sure to start easy. It is easy to overdo it in the beginning. If your solar plexus feels sore or painful later in the day, breathe deeply and circulate energy in a soft gentle way. For myself, I found that running helped, although for the first mile it would be painful. Also I found that drinking a glass of carbonated sweet drink helped. From experience, it is easy to overdue it at first without realizing it. Do not be fanatical. Properly done, the whole practice is very enjoyable and energizing.

Step Five

Get a hardwood or Raton stick. Start beating the skin, starting with the area between the navel and solar plexus and gradually extending the area. In time include the rib cage, kidneys (with caution), and shoulder blades. Start lightly and gradually increase the force. At no time should it feel painful. It is a kind of pleasurable massage. Always be sure to mentally direct prana under the area being hit, so that a feeling develops that the muscles and skin are stronger than the force of the blow. There is an actual, tangible pressure, like a balloon filled with air that absorbs the blow and energetically pushes the stick back. This is something that is gradually achieved. A quality of your aura is felt through and over the skin and muscles. If you feel a tensing, contraction, or pain under the stick, you are hitting too hard or are not yet ready to begin this part of the practice.

Before using the stick, you may want to hit with your fists. When finished, slap the skin and then smooth out the energy with gentle massage and stroking. Over time, you will be able to hit the stick quite strongly, yet it will not be painful. This is not a deadening of the area, rather you have created a lot of energy in your body that can absorb the blow and protect against it.

Gradually you develop a dual movement, where you direct a kind of penetrating energy through the stick into your body and at the same time there is a force inside your body that can both push back and absorb the energy. Between this balance you increase both the quality and quantity of energy stored in and moving through your tissues.

Additionally a bundle of wire can also be used, which supposedly can bring even further benefit as the force penetrates deeper into the organs, but I did not go this route.

Tips

After relaxing on the back for a few minutes (or more if needed), it is very advisable to quietly sit for a half-hour or longer. Circulate, soften, and absorb your energy throughout the body. Turn all your energy into soft energy. Vitalize the microcosmic orbit and other channels. Visualize the body as hollow and filled with light. This removes stagnation and deepens self-awareness beyond form. Finishing this practice with deep silent meditation is particularly fulfilling, rewarding and transforms short term benefits into long term benefits.

I found it helpful to exercise and stretch before beginning, so that I am thoroughly warmed up. Do not do so much that you are tired.

You may want to gently massage the groin area for a few minutes once or twice during the course of practice. In particular, men massage the testicles and surrounding muscles and woman the frontal mound and perhaps the breasts. This lightly stimulates sexual life-force energy, which is then drawn up to the abdominal area as you continue with the regular part of the practice. Do not create sexual eroticism or fantasy during any part of the practice, rather as sexual energy increases, feel it strengthening your body. It is thus contained and circulated as the beautiful feeling of life force. This is very important. Also, for men, be vigilant in keeping your seed during the months of practice.

I did not use the herbal formulas mentioned in Yang's book, but did use a number of various chinese herbal tonic formulas that I created for myself, which were of an overall tonifying benefit, such as shou-wu formulas.

While it is certainly nice to have someone massage you, I feel it is better to be self-dependent. In that way you will not feel you need someone else and also you will not pressure someone else when they do not feel like it. It is much easier to keep a steady practice this way (and your wrists and hands will get stronger). Then if your partner or friend wants to occasionally assist you, it is a pleasant surprise.

Remember that this practice, while a gem of great value, is not an end all. You must learn how to guide and integrate the increased energy into the various aspects of your body, and preferably use it to birth a spiritual dimension of yourself.

Fist Clenching Chi Kung

This is an abbreviation and hence one of the countless variations of a famous set of exercises given by Bodhidharma to the Shaolin Monks to help them become stronger.

While it is easy to dismiss these exercises at first glance, because they do not look like they are doing much, if done every day for several months they bring noticeable health benefits that can be described as amazing. This abbreviated practice is a simple health tonic for any person, including older people. They only take a few minutes and are enjoyable.

A practitioner who has previously developed a strong buildup of energy in the tan-tien and microcosmic orbit and is using these type of practice to expand the circulation through the arms, would practice this type of exercise more intensely than given here.

While doing these exercises there is a constant awareness of connecting energy from the hands and arms into meeting the spinal flow at the back of the heart and shoulders and then to through the microcosmic orbit. At the same time there is also a path of energy from the tan tien out through the arms. So both directions are worked with simultaneaously.

With all of these exercises, stand with feet at a comfortable distance apart and the body relaxed. Keep the back supple and straight, perhaps slightly bowed out by a fraction of an inch and the hips slightly tucked in so as to activate the kidney area. Your whole body should feel connected as you stand. Keep the mind relaxed and present.

Do each exercise for 2 to 5 minutes or count a set number of reps, for example fifty reps. For the first five exercises you may either coordinate the squeezing and relaxing of the fists with the breath or not. It is more powerful with the breath. If using the breath, then relax on the inhale and squeeze on the exhale. If you do not use the breath, then make the cycles of squeezing and relaxing a little faster.

1) Arms by sides with palms bent ninety degrees (hands stiff) pointing forward. Push the heel of the palm down. At the same time, since the hands are stiff, you will also raise the fingers up. Let the breath be relaxed and connected from the navel through to the hands. This activates an energy pump at the wrist.

2) (optional) Bring the hands into fists, bent ninety degrees at the wrist (The fists point forwards). The thumbs are separate pointing in towards the body.

3) Extend the arms straight out to each side. With the hands in fists, squeeze and relax the fists repeatedly. As you do this and the following exercises, feel energy pumped up from the wrists, start to spread and connect with the muscles and tendons of the arms, shoulders, torso, the navel and from there the whole body.

4) Keeping the upper arms out to the sides, bend at the elbows so that the fists are about six inches from the temples. Squeeze and relax the fists repeatedly.

5) Extend both arms straight out in front, shoulders relaxed down. Squeeze and relax the fists repeatedly.

6) Lower the fists so that they are a few inches from the navel or solar plexus area. The fists face each other, a few inches apart, with the palm side of the fist facing down. Tighten and squeeze them a few times. Next, totally relax the muscles (keeping the hands in fists). As you exhale mentally squeeze the fists without actually squeezing the muscles (the muscles may tense a very slight amount). As you inhale, feel the fists (and arms) totally relax, as you draw energy up the arms and through the body.

It is extremely valuable to understand how to contain and direct energy in the body. Often when people first start the practice of breathing in energy, they do not understand containment. As you exhale, direct energy through the body or within some part. As you next inhale, do not dissipate what you have already drawn in. Use part of your attention to keep the energy presence, and draw more in with the next breath to add to it. In any technique or meditation, as energy builds up in the body, it is a great health tonic to squeeze various muscles to force the energy deeper into the muscles, tendons, and the bone marrow itself. Then as your relax, feel the softness of the energy and absorb it more fully.

Sometimes energy is released from the body on the exhale to clear a channel, to remove a blockage, to release an excess, or to direct it towards another person or place. In any case, the presence of where and what the energy is doing at any time is maintained.

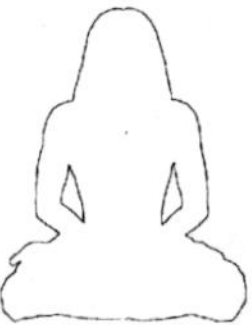

11

Chakras, Channels, Energy and Essences

This chapter details the subtle energy of our body and gives valuable techniques of exploration and discovery.

Overview

As Yoga and Tantra involves our subtle energy, it is imperative to have an understanding of our energetic aspects if we are to be successful in our practice. The energy body is a continuum that ranges from physicality to very subtle self-originating pranas that are inseparable from and simultaneously support higher consciousness. Our subtle anatomy has many variations within the fluidity of our being that make it a wonderful dance and ecstatic meditation of nectar as we awaken to our awareness.

By meditating directly on and through our subtle energy essences, we develop a natural approach to liberation, whereby the intrinsic energy within everything is divine. Whether it be trash or a flower, underneath is ecstatic life. This frees us from all dogmas and illusions, because we have found the underlying truth supporting all of existence (including our own).

Thus as you advance over the years, practice becomes simpler and more profound, truly transforming your entire perspective. The yogic art is so simple. It is not about stretching, or developing peace. Rather it is the cultivation of awareness within the core of our body in a way that develops radiant nectar, whereby we awaken into our infinity beyond and yet within our body, becoming free in pure pristine awareness itself. This is not an overnight achievement, rather a cultivation, moving in and out of apparent levels of enlightenment as simply as you change a thought, until nectar so perfumes us, that bliss drives us (meditates us) into unshakeable enlightenment.

Thus this chapter, while included in the first of this series of books, could have easily been included in the book on the higher tantras. In this book, we will focus on the realms and currents within the body. In the next book we will include the realms above the head as a shortcut method to going deeper within (a method of Eternal Yoga).

We gradually gain familiarity with our radiant body through maturity and experience, breathing, meditation, intuition, exercises and visualization. This is within the capacity of anyone who desires it, because after all, this is not something outside of us. If all the written knowledge was destroyed today and several generations passed with no written text or communication, it could all be regained through inner observance and correlation with others doing the same.

Enjoy each step of the way and understand that it often takes years for all this to gel. Connectivity is the key to working with your energy. It is more important to ground, breathe and sense than to float in an abstract image.

Our subtle energy existence can be described in terms of:

- **Channels** through which energy flows also known as Nadis, Vessels and Meridians
- The principle focal points, such as **Chakras**, otherwise known as abodes.
- **Energy** also known as Life-force, Wind, Chi, Prana and Radiance
- **Essences** such as Fluids, Drops, Nectars, Scents and Condensations of energy whereby emotional support and manifestation is given to subtle awareness.

At first, and for immediate practical application, the most important aspects to become intimate with are the major chakras in the sexual, navel, heart, throat and head areas, and the principal flows of energy in the body.

If you are just starting to become aware of the chakras, concentrate on the feeling presence and spatial awareness of their perspective areas. Think of the chakras as abodes or consciousness. When you visit a city or mountain area, go sailing on a boat, make love with your partner, ... these are all types of experiences. Just the same there are different abodes of consciousness in our body that open into realms of awareness. Some of these realms have lots of strength, or beauty or intelligence, or subtlety to them. In some, you may find yourself blending with others without limits; in others you may find yourself cherishing lots of individual definition.

Thus if all you do is focus in the area where a chakra is supposed to be, you might miss the whole experience. When you go to Hawaii, you do not dress in heavy wool coats, when you go to the high mountains in winter, you usually dress warm. To experience horses, do not pat a horse for 30 seconds and leave, rather be with them for the day, again and again. Thus when you enter an abode, go in a fashion that allows you to experience it. Hang out in it - let the quality of your inner abodes become obvious over time, not all at once. Surrender into it without preconception by lightning yourself of external pulls and abiding in the concentrated abodes of your soul essence.

While chakras may be a technical sounding and unfamiliar word, an abode is something that everyone is at least a little familiar with. An abode is a place where you live. As yogis, we are penetrating within to sit smack in the center of our form. We watch our energy becoming emotions, becoming drive, becoming everything we experience, and we can play with this, moving in and out. Life becomes fun. Life becomes heightened by holding attention grounded within, and thereby discovering the richness of our body.

As you become more familiar with the chakras, their exact centers become places where essences are cultivated and stored. The perfume and light of these essences then moves out from the center to give the whole body a fragrance of strength, beauty, bliss and many other qualities that support a refined existence. It is indescribably the feeling as we develop a consciousness that lives beyond a dense body, beyond our pettiness, that can continue both through and beyond our apparent body, that can be in several bodies, and yet lives in only one (the body of the one).

The channels are most often learned through visualizing the routes and breathing through them. The chakras are all located on and centered within energy routes or channels. Coming out of each chakra are a radiance of smaller or finer energy channels sometimes called petals, filaments or spokes. Some of these filaments in turn connect with other channels, thus creating a fluidic web throughout the body.

While there are many chakras and flows of energy in the body, a particular practice or approach most often only describes the chakras and channels relative to that practice. This creates confusion in practitioners who are looking for a set formula, because the formula keeps changing from one practice to the next. Furthermore the way the chakras are described will vary depending on what qualities of the chakra are being emphasized (or even created). Our subtle energy is something we cultivate. The potential is in everyone, yet not active in everyone. Chakras and channels are made of subtle energy, thus they wane in and out of existence according to the activation within us. In yogic practice, we learn how to give them more "substance," through the cultivation of nectar. Nectar is a magical substance. It is physical and subtle at the same time, originating beyond form and with form, coming in many flavors and expanses, beyond laws yet with great effect – it is energy and form together through the wonder of emotion, music, it is the substance of the soul.

While the basic flows and chakras are the same in everybody, there are variations in their form and expression from person to person and in the same person at different stages of development. These variations include even the existence of some subtle chakras and energy flows. If you remember that the body is an expression created by your spirit, then this should be expected. You can create a new energy flow anytime you want in the body by simply visualizing it intensely and long enough. However if there were not a good purpose for this flow, then it would naturally disappear after time.

Energy always flows, or wants to flow - it transverses all kinds of space, reveals emotion, intent and love. Soul-aware emotional-Energy bridges our mental aspect into physicality, thereby overcoming the separation of duality. When it does not flow we are stuck, when it flows, everything is fine. Tantra is the cultivation of the energy body, whereby we overcome duality in the bliss of our union.

Consciousness of any kind cannot exist without an energy that supports it. Energy and consciousness are two sides of the same coin, separate them and we live in apparent duality. This is a fundamental principle of tantra. The subtle body itself has many levels of refinement and freedom of expression. Some of these levels exist solely for the support of our physical existence and are interdependently created with it and perish with it. More refined levels of the energy body can exist on nourishment drawn from universal sources of energy and can operate as a vehicle of consciousness independent of the physical. If you work at it, this subtle energy existence can directly nourish and regenerate the physical. The most refined energy body creates its existence out of self-radiant consciousness and is thus an eternal deathless body. This radiant expression is further characterized by the degree of freedom from dualistic appearance.

It is not just a matter of discovering your subtle energy body, but to a degree, creating it. While the various levels of the body exist in everyone, few have developed themselves to anywhere near there potential. While your physical body was given its start and birth by your parents, you will birth your own dynamic and radiant existence in the Ascension process. This is the practice of Yoga, Eternal Yoga and the Higher Tantras.

THE CHAKRAS

A chakra is a focal point of subtle energy and consciousness. The principal chakras do not obey physical laws of energy conservation. Energy flows into and out of chakras, but energy can also originate or disappear, as dictated by the needs of the soul. There are hundreds of chakras within the body and each major chakra is a pivot of many smaller chakras. Chakras are like hearts.

While the chakras are subtle, not existing in physicality, our physical energy does respond to them. Without the chakras we would be dead. We can train our physical body to become more attuned to the chakras, and in so doing; physicality awakens to become an extension of our soul.

Chakras are meeting rooms where various types of experiences come together. Chakras are also drops of nectar, like the nectar within a flower. This nectar is formed, contained, refined, and available for circulation throughout the body. Because each chakra houses an image of you each chakra has its own soul quality.

To work with the chakras you must also work with the flows of energy in the body, such as the spinal, frontal and central channels. The principal chakras are places along these channels. The flows are the reality of all the chakras being of one energy-form. Going with the flow is wonderful and necessary and yet if that is all you do, this will not reveal its inner origination. For this you must enter deep into the chakras from which the flows originate. This inner penetration reveals the flow of life itself. The sense of one big chakra comes into a stronger feeling when the eighth center above the head is activated and grounded into bodily awareness. This is the place where all the bodily chakras are initially patterned. The eighth center will be explored in the next book in this series, when we open up the subject of Eternal Yoga.

A chakra is an amazing wheel of energy with several layers and manifestations of its existence. The major chakras all have filaments of energy that connect to other chakras, the energy space of an organ, various areas of the body, or sometimes through inner space to a particular being, location, or realm. At first you can ignore these energetic lines and simply concentrate on the sense of presence and inner space in the area of the chakra itself. Later on, it is important to experience the fullness of the chakra in its expression and outreach.

The major chakras are all centered within the principal flows of energy through the body. Depending on how you are centering within the chakra, which of these flows a chakra is centered in can appear to change. This is not an ambiguity, but the spatial nature of the deeper realms themselves and the multi-facetted aspects of the chakras. For example the spinal chakras are all centered within the spinal column. However, upon going deeper into the chakra the centering changes to the central (fusion) channel (which is internal to the spine,) and a filament connects to the spinal flow from the chakra.

Various descriptions and systems may describe the number of petals from each chakra differently. Again, this is reflective of how those chakras are being used and the amount of detail that each system feels is sufficient. There is a vast possibility of energy interconnection within each of us and out of that possibility certain connections are brought forth and others (from a level of focus) are ignored.

While the chakras are subtle (not visible to most people), nonetheless, they are actual and tangible places. Some of the nectar produced by the endocrine glands binds with and receives subtle energy from the chakras. By activating the chakras we stimulate the gland and at the same time help contain and refine these secretions within the body. This is one of ways of uniting presence with matter, thereby developing both. The most important of these secretions are the sexual fluids.

As you start to get a feeling for the location of the chakras, feel your presence emanating out of the chakras into your body and the space around you. Since the outer aspects of the chakras are intertwined with our physiology, the outer aspects of the chakras are relatively easy to sense and work with. The inner aspects require much more sensitivity and grounding. The definition gained by going within the chakras is a vital part of creating the inner temple.

Many describe the chakras as spinning vortexes. This is a way of working with the outer aspects of the chakras. However, for myself, this does not give any connection to, or accurate reflection of, the inner heart of a chakra or its structure. A technique that arose from within me for entering the inner heart of a chakra is to first vitalize the flows of energy connected to that chakra through breathing and visualization, and then to enter into the center of it. This requires a firm inner placement of attention and steady mind. Once there, I feel myself drawing all the energy of my body inwards into an area about a quarter inch in diameter of which I am centered within. There is an immediate feedback of an effortless bliss as my prana enters into the center and sometimes a loss of regular bodily awareness as the consciousness is absorbed into that inner world. When centering within, a huge space opens up. As you become familiar with that inner space you can reverse the process and thereby bring about a greater integration of body and mind.

The above technique is somewhat advanced and should only be employed in earnest after you have become familiar with the major chakras and energy flows of the body. A whole body feeling should already be natural along with a sense of positive radiance most of the time. If your mind and energy level becomes dull or sleepy while trying the above it is reflective that you are not centered enough within the chakra, there is not enough vitality to serve the transition, or that there are blockages within the energy-channels connected to that chakra. In this case you should continue general breathing within the body, visualization of the chakras and energy routes, and a positive radiant feeling from the inside out. Physical exercise also helps. Another reason to have already established yourself in the whole body feeling is so that you do not become too introverted and disconnected when doing techniques such as above.

Some methods use the visualization of a symbol or letter within each chakra that is connected to a sound (mantra). This is an aid to better focus. Your mind becomes one with that symbol and takes its form, which emanates a sound (prana) and quality (of consciousness). The symbol is a way of maintaining concentration and for many people is an excellent approach. The only drawback is if the symbol, because of a lack of completeness in application, creates a sense of separation through a mechanical quality of the universe. In other words, it is not you. The other consideration of this approach is that it often requires an inner transmission (initiation) to really get the feel of it. For example, the sound "Ahh," often used as an expression of the energy body, if concentrated upon as a sort of emotionless flat sound, does not give the proper sense of connectivity. It was not until Mahavatar BabaJi came in a dream, transformed himself into the sound of "Ah," entered within my heart, and became me as that sound, that I emotionally and energetically understood its power and totality. It has the release, absorption, emotional-movement and ecstasy of the "Ahh" of making Love and yet at the same time the sound could continue without a break in breath or cycle.

Another example is the sound of "Hum." If you just say Hum all day, well, so what. Rather that Hum needs to be connected to a very fine stream of all-encompassing effortless prana (a subtle body) that constantly radiates out its existence from within the heart. You can meditate on this subtle body just fine, if you so choose, without the sound of Hum. However if before understanding this subtle body, you blindly try to use the sound of Hum to connect with it, you are going about things backwards. The sound of Hum is a way of maintaining awareness, or it is one of the elements acting as a carrier of prana to help that penetration of awareness.

Do not blindly follow technique; rather strive for the alive inner feeling. By so doing you will connect and receive further support from an inner level. Mahavatar BabaJi (also known as Padmasambhava) stresses to me the importance of connectivity and not making shortcuts. As an example; if I am doing a technique of moving energy up and down the spine, if there is a persistent blind area or blockage, I will stop my technique and instead focus there and the surrounding tissues, breathe through it, see what I need to see and correct it. Often it is just about getting more grounded in that area or aspect. Then I can again take up the original technique, which is now many times more effective. However, if I do not give myself permission to deviate from the technique, then this could never occur, and I am taking a rather slow route.

The chakras described here are the ones most often used in developing the energy body, which of course includes the physical, emotional and mental qualities. While each chakra has its own flavor, if all the chakras are felt as part of one big chakra, then that center is from within the heart. Some may feel that this center is in the head instead because of the tremendous expansiveness and transcendence. However, as you go further, above the head, it eventually returns full circle, and once again centers within the heart. This occurs as the innermost space of the heart is spatially at one with all the other centers above, below, within and without.

Base of the Spine

Opening the base of your spine is being happy and vital here on planet earth. It has been called the key to enlightenment within some Taoist teachings and the Tibetan tantras call it "the secret place."

Working with earth energies requires this opening. The simplest way to begin is to work with the flow of energy. Inhale down the front of your body, underneath, and exhale your precious prana up through the tailbone. A common mistake is to keep the energy too close to the surface of the skin. Concentrate on a warm pathway about an inch or more under the skin (within the bone marrow).

The base of the spine is very connected to the perineum, one of the major energy collection points lying halfway between the genitals and anus. You can collect energy here to build it before sending it up through the tailbone. As you direct and visualize energy through the tailbone, move slowly and with a thick sensation. As a warm opening sensation occurs, do not let it slip away while inhaling and gentle increase the sensations with each exhale. Slowly, like a light made out of molasses, guide it up the tailbone and spine. Once it reaches the vertebrae, it can be moved upwards easily and more quickly with the breath and attention.

You may want to practice lying in bed first thing in the morning or if your wake up during the night. Start by breathing through the feet to energize them. Then continue up through the ankles, the inside of the legs, and finally vitalizing the perineum. Take at least five or ten minutes with just your feet. Next breathe down the frontal line, combine the energy at the perineum, and then start up the tailbone. As the energy moves up the spine, energize the kidneys. This gives a feeling of potent containment and strength. Lying in bed doing this breathing is also a good way to relieve tiredness.

If the breathing results in a sexual stimulation but no opening of the tailbone area, then keep breathing and allow that stimulation for five minutes or so. Next, inhale and hold the breath while contracting the genitals inwards and then squeeze the anus tightly. You want to squeeze the muscles of the anus not just at its opening, but also several inches up the rectum. This is a key. Hold for about twenty seconds and then exhale, being conscious to exhale up through the tailbone and in this case at least up to the kidneys. Do this several times. Then relax and work with the energy very softly and pleasantly. Squeezing the anus like this is also an excellent health tonic.

Martial arts stances help open the base of the spine. When this practice becomes proficient, the tailbone will often realign and move or click into place within five to fifteen minutes of beginning the practice.

Concentrating at the base of the spine and the perineum increases the earth element in your body. The base of the spine has a natural polarity with the crown chakra and also strengthens the heart area. These three chakras are all seats of the astral body, which is a term for your emotional nonverbal being. These chakras are also gateways into physical, subtle, and very subtle modes of existence.

When you are ready to start focusing within the base of the spine chakra also known as mhuladhara, connect with an area about an inch across in the spine an inch and a half to two inches above the very tip of the tailbone. Visualize this chakra as a bright, earthy blood red. Yellow or White are alternative colors that also work well in this chakra. If using red, it is not composed of fire but of an earthy connectivity.

Let the light of this chakra light up this area of your body with a presence moving up into the whole body and sense that it connects to realms within the earth. The base chakra stores a lot of imprints from social conditioning. Thus it is a good place to free some of this conditioning. When doing so, bring in a guiding hand from the crown and heart centers. Many images can be seen within the light of this chakra, and by seeing them you gain insight and the ability to change them if so desired. If you do not have a sense of intimacy within yourself, it is likely that you will shut down the vision within this chakra.

Energizing this chakra will create greater ease of movement. It gives a greater sense of security. Worldly pressures, such as finances, concern about reputation, etc., have less power to move you out of your center. The light from this chakra makes the body feel more transparent. In this transparency, it is easier to connect to the sense that you are part of a omniscient power at work in the physical.

Sexual

When the sexual center is referred to as a chakra it is usually in reference to the spinal chakra about halfway between the base of the spine and opposite the navel It is also commonly called the second chakra. However, there are a number of energy centers that are part of our sexuality and sometime when a person is referring to the sexual chakra they mean the perineum, base of the spine chakra, and various parts of or areas connected to the genitals including the lower frontal line.

The second spinal chakra is very connected to the throat center and the eighth center just above the crown. This is because all these chakras are principally concerned with the etheric structure also known as the energy body. As liquid light, the life force through the first and second chakras connects with and is drawn up by an activation of any of the spinal centers. The sexual nectars as they are refined and collected in the back of the head, throughout the head in general, the forehead, the thymus and heart area for the yogi or yogini bring a connection between our sexuality and these areas. It is even possible to experience an orgasmic response in these areas through sexual embrace and increase, which is truly a feeling you will never forget.

When the energy "cracks" open or penetrates into the second chakra within the spinal marrow it is an incredible blissful, light, implosive, mystical and passionate feeling. However getting the energy into the marrow of the spine where this opening occurs often requires a filling out of all the earth chakras and area below the navel first. This includes the perineum, genitals, base of the spine, kidneys, tan-tien (a point on the front just below the navel), and the pubic bone area. That means feeling a lot of sexual energy and being able to just be with it, while refining and directing it inwards and upwards.

To get this energy into and through the tailbone often require that we bring the prana of our breath down to this area to mix with the energy and help it upwards. Simply breathing and visualizing our energy down the sides of the spine into the tailbone and then up through the spine itself helps to bring this about, combined with a polarized draw from the third eye. Once we enter into the tailbone, we need to bring it into the command of the navel area to keep the momentum upwards. The microcosmic orbit introduced later in this chapter also greatly helps this penetration and movement and can be used as the primary method of getting the energy through this part of the pathway.

Sexual energy moves up the body a number of ways. It moves through the organs, blood, lymph and connective tissues. As an energy-substance-feeling it is moved through the spinal marrow, frontal line and/or the inside of the legs. A more advanced practice is to bring some or almost all of the energy up through the central channel. When the central channel is engaged, then tantric consort practice from a perspective of higher enlightenment becomes a possibility. At this point there are mystical chakras within the genitals themselves that become very important in helping to create the tantric (nectar) body.

Refined sexual energy is not an explosive wanting relief type of activity. It is life force itself and this grosser idea of it must be gradually burned out through experience and refinement. Before exploring the second chakra by focusing there in meditation you should have already become familiar with some of the major energy routes of the body and the upper chakras.

The second chakra has a strong connection with the water element, the kidneys and your bones. The kidneys are a storehouse and generator of sexual potency. The feeling essence and support of the kidneys are essential to generate subtle nectars that ground "feeling" light within the body. The kidneys mostly work with the water element combined with earth and some fire. This combination when brought into the navel point with a sensual feeling and contained there ignites a kind of mystical water-fire, stabilized through a very fine oil-like medium that is tremendously nourishing to the inner spaces of the body. The natural quality of the kidneys is containment of energy.

The Taoists talk about the kidneys containing the original essence from our parents and when this is consumed, we die. I believe this "original jing" is our body blueprint, our DNA and similar mechanisms of defining form and constitution. The kidneys are the soul of the lifeforce that maintains and repairs the DNA, so that it may act as an antenna to the subtle lifeforce of our finer bodies, thereby grounding its form and energy. The DNA according to scientific study has many functions in acting as the template by which RNA creates the countless proteins necessary to maintain life. Again, without this energy our cellular blueprint cannot repair and maintain itself.

The water quality of our sexuality is absolutely necessary to balance the fire of our meditative effort and mind if we are to achieve a continuum of spirit and form. Later in this chapter will be introduced the central channel through which we create our inner temple. Because the primary conducive element of the central channel is its water quality, at least to start with, this is a reason that sexual energy is so often referred to and used as a means to ignite the spiritual bliss and awareness of the central channel. However this is unlikely to occur with any real effect unless the central channel is first very familiar to us, otherwise our energy goes elsewhere and everywhere.

A feeling of wanting sexual release can be created through agitation or toxicity in the liver. If energy is expelled in this way, instead of circulating the energy, of course it weakens the body. A good diet, exercise and emotional clarity keeps the liver clean. The liver contains our self-images, and if our sexual images include an outward expulsion of energy then those images become manifest in the body.

Thus creating a passionate, yet contained sexual helps to manifest this containment. Without this, there is no way that our sexual energy can be integrated as a source of power and fluidity into our whole being. Look at a classical Tibetan picture of a divine couple making love (called a yub-yam). If you are a man, then feel the intercourse, and within your body you will notice one of two responses, both of which are sensual in nature. Either your energy wants to go out and into the woman, or it moves upwards in a sense of strength and passion, which can then be shared with the woman through your entire being. When you look at the image, feel the man containing that energy of shakti and you will understand. It is this image you want to cultivate, not one of release. This requires refinement and internalization, both of which are feminine in nature. Thus a man must embrace his feminine aspect to integrate his sexual energy, and to be a good lover.

For a woman, there has to be an image of ecstatic deepening, not one of needing the energy on a superficial level. This is not to deny that energy is needed on an external level, but that it is only a small part of the bigger equation. While the magic word for a man is containment, which opens the doors for him, for a woman it is making love with divinity, which is both in her and outside of her. If the woman feels too much that she is needing to be filled up, then this externalizes the energy in a subtle way that prevents its opening within the deeper spaces, which is necessary for the divine fulfillment of sexual energy.

Navel and Tan Tien

The navel area is an important kingdom that prepares earth to mix with heaven. More than any other area of the body, the navel region can take in large amounts of prana and assimilate it as a force to refine and energize our body. If properly qualified and directed this amounts to a spiritual dynamo.

The navel energy is the field director that has the strength to mix with the seduction of sexuality and say, "this way." However, this field director needs to be seduced by the heart and a deeper level of being. You must be careful with how you seduce your navel. If it takes to bed flagrant emotion you become unstable. If, as brain, it sides with the rational mind, it can be outwardly efficient, yet, from a spiritual perspective constantly get in its own way. Rather the navel presence must become a natural aspect of your grounded spiritual being; flexible, empowered, surrendered, transparent and part of a whole body feeling.

The navel functions to nourish and more specifically to assimilate nourishment into something your body can use. The navel is a power area lit by fire. If this fire is to rejuvenate then it must include moisture, movement and inner surrender. Without vitality of the navel and what it commands spiritual development of the physical body is only a fantasy.

Navel exercises and massage clears the organs and vitalizes the connective tissues. This helps to develop a good spatial sense of that area of your body, which is necessary to gain firmness in holding concentration upon the heart of the navel chakra.

The navel area encompasses a number of closely connected chakras, principally the navel center, tan-tien, and solar plexus. The navel area may be developed through any of these chakras, and development of one links to the others. The navel chakra is half way between the sides of the body and more towards the back than the front. Some people experience the center a little above or a little below the level of the navel. From this center are many filaments of energy spreading out horizontally like the spokes of a wheel, each connecting to various functions of the body. When it comes time to enter the center of this chakra, then working with at least some of these filaments helps maintain the firm focus within the center. This is a result of symmetry, one of the most important principles of developing the inner temple.

For the purpose of symmetry, the filaments of the four directions are most important and if your use eight directions, that is better. From the navel center there is a filament that connects to the spinal (surface) chakra in the rear, the frontal line in the front, and to each of the side channels of the vertical channels. If you are using eight or more filaments then connect some of them to the kidneys, some of them to each side of the navel and the rest of them intuit as connecting to every area of the body. These side filaments after connecting to the vertical channels continue onwards to connect to the sides of the body and organ energy. Visualize the filaments, as small tubes that are flexible and soft and filled with a blood like oily nectar. You can visualize additional filaments (the Tibetan system uses 64 of them). Like a large flower, it forms a canopy that collects fragrance from the heart and lungs. Energy coming in and out through these filaments or petals of the flower heals and energizes the entire body, just like a light bulb lights a room and a fire warms it.

The center of the chakra is only about the size of a marble, although you can use a sphere as large as three inches to start with or to help connect the chakra with your organ energy. Within the center lives a cosmic fire. If you bring the essence of your blood and your seminal fluids to this center then an amazing connectivity to your body results through that medium.

The navel chakra is not the same as the navel point. The navel point lies on the frontal line, while the navel chakra lies towards the spine. Entering the heart of the navel chakra is actually a fairly advanced practice and for a beginning practitioner is a future event.

Breathing and visualization techniques to gather, concentrate and mix large amounts of energy are only safe at the navel area. If for example, this was done at the heart serious health complications and even danger to life can result. Of course for very advanced adepts, other centers can be safely cultivated (and sometimes are) for this type of mixing, but why not use the natural ability of the navel for this. The other centers then take this already refined energy and gently mix it for an even more sublime expression of the soul. An example would be the mixing of experience and emptiness within the heart or the mixing of various nectars within the heart to support entering the eternal light of consciousness. Very large amounts of energy can be mixed through the crown center, but this is an advanced esoteric practice only within the scope of one who is truly ready.

General yoga sets given in this book help to purify and enliven the navel area. Vase breathing techniques given in this book (in the inner-fire practice) introduce the adept to awakening the kundalini of the navel, and are best done under the guidance of a teacher in coordination with other aspects of the spiritual path. Gently visualizing and focusing nectar like light and brightness with centered breathing within the navel as "part of" your practice is a relatively safe and good means to gradually open your navel center.

The chakras are not in the physical body, yet have a play into the physical through the continuum of our being. Thus it is possible for different individuals, and the same individual at different time, to ground the same chakra into the body in slightly different places. This is perhaps most evident in the navel center. Also keep in mind that different aspects of a chakra can be grounded into different, yet similar places in the body.

In the case of the navel center, its grounding at that level of the navel point has a greater fire quality, while sinking its grounding a few inches below the navel gives it a greater support of the water element. Likewise grounding it deeper into the body gives it a greater water quality and support, while relating to the navel chakra closer to the front or the back of the spine results in a weaker and inconsistent relationship into the physical.

Because a practitioner either instinctually goes to particular areas or is taught to do so, that practitioner will say the navel chakra is in this place or that.

The Tan Tien is on the frontal line approximately one and a half inches below the navel and a few inches inward. Yet it can also refer to a sinking of the navel chakra, in which case it is closer to the spine. This sinking of the navel chakra, helps the navel energy to better mix with the sexual energy, thereby moistening it and increasing its passion.

For some this deeper aspect of the TanTien may be felt as a mixing of the second and third chakras while for others it is the third chakra itself. Both experiences are valid.

The tan-tien (frontal point) is capable of gathering and focusing a lot of energy that can then be directed inwards towards the spine, for deeper assimilation by the body and for spiritual vitalization.

The Tan Tien brings the genital, kidney and navel expressions all together and thus creates an inner space between these three places whereby a quality of the self can be nourished. The tan tien is a very intimate center. To really experience a deep permanent sense of the tan tien that energizes you throughout the day then learn to feel it deep in the body. The surface aspect of it is simply to collect energy from the kidneys and organs which is then led into its deeper aspect.

By emphasizing the tan-tien rather than the navel you connect with more nourishment from the lower chakras, which bring in a watery and earth element. This is important for balance and health. Because of a better water-fire balance, in some practices the tan-tien is often emphasized more than the navel. Yet what aspect of the tan-tein you are using, the frontal line, or spinal sinking of the navel chakra creates a very different flavor. Practitioners gravitate towards the various chakras of the navel region depending on their constitution, what they need elementally, what type of energy they are focusing thorough in the moment, and what dimensional-aspects of their being they are working with in that moment.

Rather than listing the advantages or disadvantages of choosing one particular point of focus over another, this is something best realized through each persons experience over the years. Some rules of thumb; the frontal line initially is better for creating vitality. The spinal line is better for command of and raising of the energy, and the ecstatic deep mixing of the front and back on the center, towards the spine is what is developed through maturity of practice. Slightly above or at the level of the navel point is more of rational, mental, driven male fire energy, while sinking down a bit is more a fluid passionate intimate feminine blending energy.

The Tan Tien can absorb a lot of energy from your environment. With certain activations of the silver ray from above the head deep into the body, I have experienced a subtle beam of energy that projects out for hundreds of feet from the tan tien. The silver ray is a high stakes and very free vehicle of awareness and through it a being can either entrap their self or enter into a greater expression of their cosmic self.

Solar Plexus

The solar plexus is not really a primary chakra, although it can become one if the navel chakra gets its primary grounding into this part of the body[1]. Rather the solar plexus is one of the premier mixing places of energy and essences in the body to bring forth a lot of physically and subtly felt presence. The solar plexus is a place of power, transmutation and projection of earthly command. It is a good place to clothe subtle presence through visualization. It is a place of manifestation through creative visualization. The solar plexus often has a white or a golden energy to it.

The Solar Plexus is an inner space whereby an intermediate energy body can soar on wings of freedom through the astral realms. The astral realms are composed of emotional-dream-like-substance. One has to be careful that the great confidence the solar plexus instills does not overtake humility and compassion.

The upper part of the solar plexus is the lower orb of the heart chakra. This orb contains memory of the many people who you have emotional interacted with over many lifetimes. The lower part of the solar plexus is a refined aspect of the navel energy.

Advanced practices whose aim is to create an eternal consciousness in the buddhic realms often ignore the solar plexus. If you want to create a fully conscious expression here in the physical then you need to integrate the solar.

The solar plexus is a place to see, be present and take command or at least to wrestle with the forces of command. Successful businessmen and woman as a general rule have a well-developed presence within the solar plexus and much of their subtle communication with each other occurs from this place.

1 In my opinion it is not advisable to make the solar plexus the primary grounding of the navel chakra, as it will not receive its full energy this way and may cause some problems of too much upward floating energy. Rather develop the navel chakra at the navel or tan-tien height and then bring up the energy into the solar plexus.

Breathing through and clearing blockages of the solar plexus is important for self-empowerment. Often in this clearing, desires of what you want or need for yourself come to light. This often terminates relationships that get in the way of this fulfillment and thus it takes a lot of courage to look within this light and see what you want. My advice is upon discovering your own hidden desires that before jumping the gun, take the time for those desires to have audience with love and your highest wisdom. Do not let theses desires take total control of your whole being and yet do not ignore them either. In this way your excitement serves you. Otherwise, the fatal spiritual mistake happens whereby you identify with the outer expression as yourself. You cannot walk, run, fly, row, crawl, giveaway, demand, follow or transport yourself to ultimate spiritual awareness. It is not something that can be achieved through ambition, goals or imagination. Rather, it is a natural state of underlying awareness within everything that has a good home within the heart.

The solar plexus gives courage. In reality there is only one relationship and that is with divinity. Without this understanding tantra never really happens, because emotional attachment gets in the way and confuses the view of emptiness and form as one. This clarity is the birthplace of effortless courage.

Rather than condense the solar plexus into a small area keep it fairly expanded. This is consistent with its mixing and refining function. Three or four inches in diameter is a good size to focus within. Prana from the diaphragm, the imaging power of the liver, the earthy tangible golden-white light of the spleen and the presence of the kidneys all surround this space. Consciously drawing in these energies adds to the solar plexus experience.

This is a place to clothe your subtle body with substance, and simultaneously it is a place to nourish your physical.

The Heart and its Kingdom

The heart chakra is our heart of hearts. Love is all you need… The heart is the supreme mixing ground of heaven and earth, being well endowed with both qualities.

The heart chakra is a vast kingdom of energy-substance grounded through nonverbal eloquence. The heart when entered is complete and yet if above and below are not complete, it is not complete. A song that cannot be sung is not yet complete.

The center of the heart chakra is between the nipples and halfway between your front and back (a little more to the back). The temple of the heart is an orb of energy approximately three to five inches in diameter, while the center of it is about the size of pea to the size of a golf ball depending on the frame of reference and how you are entering it. Most of the time it is the size of a marble. When you are cognizant of that center a peaceful balance is felt undisturbed by the distant waves of life's dramas.

Within the heart there are literally worlds upon worlds. For some the heart is mushy, romantic, forgiving, and/or capable of feeling jealousy, attachment and insecurity. For some it is a ground of adventure and for all of us, in various degrees of awareness, it is the home of the eternal presence within our body. Within the heart is the unification of all space, above and below as one. The heart contains the end of separation as an illusion. This is the delicate balance achieved through meditation and right livelihood.

The heart chakra has within it a seat of consciousness called clear light that continually radiates. The form this light takes is your eternal existence and the qualities of this light are your soul characteristics. Entering into the center of the heart is a gateway beyond the world of duality and karma. This gateway is the same as what I call the tenth realm far above the head.

When I first started to become aware of the realms above the head (in 1984), I instinctively started working with the symmetrical alignment of how they were grounding into my body. A being in a pitch black body which could not be seen started to help me prepare to enter into a place of which he said there was no turning back. This place was far above the head and very subtle. He would give me lots of tests to see how I would handle various situations. As this was occurring, for about a year, I slowly became aware of a sphere within the center of my heart a little less than an inch in diameter. It was like a black hole and this startled me. Around this sphere were other spheres. Those surrounding spheres always had lots of movement and subtle activity within them. These outer spheres were causative subtle realms that connected all the way into the physical. The inner sphere seemed to be totally still, and I could enter it half/half, but I was not ready to fully plunge into it. At the time, it was not comfortable for me to meditate on the color black, and this whole awareness was not something that I invoked, but simply happened. Thus the year of preparation was in part simply getting comfortable with going into this unknown.

As everything was aligned from above the head into the heart and the awareness of the spheres became more stable, I entered into that black hole. The entire universe disappeared into a black light of no boundary or center. It was beyond sleep, and in that I remained conscious. Gradually, in that blackness appeared forms of a light that is beyond light. This blackness is more than the blackness of outer space. It is the potential, the emptiness in which everything exists (this is different than the black-light of matter). This light was whatever my consciousness was. Anything that I saw and judged, I would become, yet it was not a problem, because the basic nature of everything was understood. That is why I call it the gateway of purity.

This awareness has never gone away. If another has that penetration into the heart, it can be seen, and it is from this place that the twin-ray is understood. For those who say there is no individual soul, I say there is, and for those who claim the separation of soul, I say there is not. This is enlightenment and it is only a beginning of which there is no end.

Long meditation within the heart is not recommended for the beginner. This can result in too much energy being focused within the physical heart tissues, an undesirable condition that can be dangerous to your health. The actual entrance into the heart is small and it is not about brute force, rather a refined delicacy, openness, fluidity and stability. In entering the heart chakra you must first train your bodies energy to maintain its natural balance and circulation while you concentrate in the heart with a subtle mind. This is also a training in how to use the mind in this manner. Otherwise your grosser energies will follow your mind into the heart center and disrupt the heart by focussing too much energy within it. Exercise and balanced meditation techniques create a whole body sense of which the heart is naturally present. Within this precious body of yours, slowly and consistently become familiar with the inner temple and it's blissful flow. Become a yogi or yogini. Through the years of consistent practice, the heart will come forth as the place to mix heaven and earth to birth what is eternal, as your presence so embraced.

There are eight filaments that come horizontally in and out of the heart chakra. These eight filaments allow a royal court of mastery to be present, so that the heart may hold majesty. One filament goes to the back, connecting to the spinal marrow and that outpouring. One goes to the front and the heart's forward projection. One goes to each side, which in turn spirals around the heart in joy. One goes to the front-left side of the heart and one to the front-right side from which demigods sometimes sit in self-proclaimed importance. One goes to each side of the back of the heart bringing healing and acceptance. If these spokes are felt to form a round table of which sits enlightened presence, then that presence blesses the penetration into the heart, removes subtle obstructions from the higher realms and becomes the bearers of its good news.

In addition to these horizontal filaments, there is an intimate upward connection to the thymus, which is a residence of freedom. Below, it connects to the solar plexus and its earthly prana.

Keep the eight spokes connected to their directions within the body, while also mixing heaven and earth from above and below. Make theses filaments small hollow flexible tubes and shine light within them. These tubes continue to their destination and in reality branch again and again to interconnect through the whole body like capillaries. On each tube a few inches out from the center sense and visualize an enlightened presence. Invite the Ascended Host to take seat within those places or sense that they are there. Do not let this whole affair float like a spaceship, but keep it connected to the body's physiology. Use that support to enter the innermost chambers of the heart and let the heart come out through that wheel of life. This wheel creates the symmetry around the heart. Through symmetry of the energy body, the higher openings are stabilized. This is a great esoteric secret that when combined with the flows of the inner temple brings liberation and tantric blending of all our many aspects.

There are also systems using 10, 12, 14 and 16 spokes. These are all valid and reflect different nuances of the heart chakra. For example by including the central channel, i.e., up and down our 8 spokes become 10. This is simply a difference in semantics. The heart chakra maybe felt to cup either upwards, downwards or both. By duplicating the NE, NW, SE and SW spokes, i.e., one curving slightly up and one curving slightly down we have 12 spokes. By including the up and down through the central channel we have 14 spokes. There are also other systems and other ways of relating to the subtle anatomy of the heart chakra, some of which do not use spokes at all.

Thymus

The thymus center is an entryway into the inner earth. It has a special connection to the central channel running up through the center of the body. The thymus sits atop the heart and is energetically half way between the heart and the throat centers. When activated it promotes a lot of etheric activity.

When I first started my yogic practices I thought the heart chakra was at the thymus. It actually took me a few years for this conviction to sink down into the actual heart center. The thymus chakra is what I call the inner earth heart and is often developed in Devic beings. It has a certain type of detachment to it with a sense of a floating freedom combined with an altruistic nature. A centering in the thymus can create naivety. Through greater penetration, willingness to see, grounding, and tantric blending this naivety disappears.

A young child has a lot of activity around the pineal gland. In growing older the pineal shrinks and much of this activity shifts to the thymus. After puberty the thymus starts to shrink as the genital area becomes more activated. In the process of rejuvenation, the energy is returned back up, revitalizing the thymus and then the pineal. In this upward turn the genitals remain active. It is not enough for the energy to simply cycle back up through the body, as it must carry with it your mastery and growing awareness.

As sweet nectars drip down from the head into the body, they should collect at each of the chakras. As they collect at the thymus gland area, there is a lot of rejuvenating benefits to the body.

The Throat Center

The throat chakra, along with the sexual and thymus chakras are the principal seats of the etheric body. The etheric body is another term for the form aspect of our energy body. Think of the etheric body as a kind of template around which energy-substance gathers and gives greater expression to, similar to the way that emotion gathers around an idea to give it expression. The etheric body is simply a more refined version of our physical body in many ways. There is a lot of energy available in the universe, but without a form for it to take, it will not be our experience.

The throat gives not just vibratory direction, but when turned inward presents an experience of bliss. In this way it is a teacher for the rest of the body. While this inward mixing can be first experienced at any center, the throat chakra is one of the easiest places to do this, because of the close proximity of various types of energy within the throat, and the easy ability to create a meditative spatial sense within the throat center. In addition the throat naturally has an impersonal, detached disposition that makes it easier to hold a pure energetic focus.

By symmetrically filling out the throat chakra with your presence much needless telepathic chatter can be overcome and thoughts pacified. When entered with enough intensity, consuming intense bliss is, as previously mentioned, experienced.

The throat center is a principle seat of the dream body. By concentrating within it lucidity and quantity of dreams are increased. Through taking command in the throat center fifth dimensional mischief-makers, power abusers, and phenomenal or curiosity seekers will not be able to disturb your meditation (or activities).

Until the throat center is somewhat activated, there is not the energetic-support in the body to sit for longer periods of time. Rather, after a half-hour to an hour the attention wanders or gets sleepy. When the throat center becomes active and clear, then a subtle energy supports the body to sit for longer times, and it is easier to stay awake within that.

Kundalini cannot be stabilized in your body without opening the throat chakra and the subtle command of harmony through it. Meditating in the throat chakra helps to, at least temporarily, overcome doubt.

The throat chakra collects nectars from the head and retains them so that they can be absorbed and distributed to the rest of the body. If these nectars are not retained for a while, then they will tend to dissipate quickly to the outer chakras and simply evaporate. In this way the throat chakra has a special relationship with the head centers.

The throat center helps an understanding of subtly and to comprehend what people are saying underneath their actual words. The throat center also, obviously, has much to do with communication. It is a center of movement and affects the body's metabolism. The throat chakra brings expansion and the sense of space.

The Tibetan Buddhist Tantras talk of sixteen filaments from this chakra and I have found it advantageous to connect with all sixteen of them. These filaments extend out horizontally like spokes of a wheel and then further divide and spread out through the body. They can be visualized as a net to catch nectar dripping down from the head into the throat where the nectar is retained for awhile.

A fun visualization is to sit as a master within the center of the throat and imagine miniature "Oms" (English letters are fine) an inch out from the center on each filament, each on fire with their radiance. For most of us, it takes a number of sittings to accomplish this, so be patient. The Oms are vibrating the sound "Om" like teenagers alive with energy, barely able to contain all their enthusiasm, vitality and potential, yet seduced by the depth of this experience. It is feeling-energy vibrating the fabric of creation as the fabric of creation, not dependent on the particular accent or variation in which you pronounce the sound "Om."

Imagine a deep blissful sound rumbling through your body, it is the rumbling, the energy, and the sensual-vibration deep inside. Try to tell someone what the sound of rumbling is without using any reference to feeling or spatial connectivity or direct-knowing. This is what is its like to give a mantra to someone just as letters on a page. It is way beyond any particular sound expressed through physical language, rather the physical language sound is just a starting point, an entryway and one of many possible gateways.

While the throat center can be stimulated in ten minutes, to really enter the throat chakra requires a an hour or two of meditation. Entering this chakra is an enjoyable experience.

Overview of the Head Chakras

There are many chakras in and around the head that all interconnect. Thus the opening of one of these chakras is often, in reality the opening of several of them working together. There is a tremendous fluidity in the nature of these interconnections that enhances intelligence and skillful means.

The head chakras are like a machine that comes to a grinding halt when no oil is present. This oil originates primarily from the refined sexual chemistry of the body. Overusing the head, without this oil, is like running a motor without oil; it burns up. When this oil is present it changes the whole nature of the head chakras from one of intellectuality, abstraction, self-absorption and ignorance to cosmic beauty. Furthermore this machine requiring oil, when working properly, makes more nectar-oil that flows through the body, which is an ecstatic experience. It is possible to live on these nectars without any intake of regular food; everyone gets some nourishment this way.

If you are quiet, various sounds can be heard within the head, which are produced by the movement of fluids and the flow of various energies (prana). Listening to these sounds can be a way of helping to maintain focus, and by resting in the more delicate sounds we can learn to center into a very subtle spacious energy of consciousness from which these sounds originate.

Toxins from dense food and too much thinking creates a residual substance that interferes with the higher capacity of the brain to receive subtle energy. Constant intellectuality, more than anything else, interferes with this capacity by making an actual chemical residue in the brain that reinforces separation. When thoughts are constantly bringing your attention away from your nonverbal center, how can the cosmic chemistry ever happen?

Center of the Head and Crown

The center of the head mixes and coordinates energy drawn in through the various head chakras and has a direct relationship with the pineal gland. The center of the head is the aspect of the crown chakra that is more bodily orientated. The pineal gland helps us to be crystal clear, symmetrically balanced with a keen discernment.

The aspect of the crown chakra near the skull is a gateway to energies and your existence outside of your physical-energy space. If you want to connect with the Ascended Masters, or with anyone that has developed a presence in the budhic realms, then open your crown chakra. Simply focusing at the top of the head with an open feeling and swirling an energy through it that includes the area just above and just inside the skull most easily does this. Simultaneously opening the palms of the hands and soles of the feet makes it easier, and brings a better integration as well. Opening the crown chakra lead directly into the area above the head which is a subject of Eternal Yoga.

You can bring healing to the body by sensing the top part of the brain as a mass of light substance with multicolored sparkles that is reflected down into the body. Within this golden light in the top portion of your head, see any area of the body that needs healing as an image of light that is vibrant, bright, and feels good. Sense that part of the body responding to this image, and a resonant bidirectional current between the top of your head and that part of the body.

When meditating in your head centers is no longer a mental, spacey, or disconnected experience, but an indescribable mix of nourishing seductive nectar, infinite space and a heart-like quality, then your head gains the capacity to mix very large amounts of cosmic energy-presence into the body. A definite sense that we are more than our individual identity is very strong. We can experience a state beyond the body and a deep effortless grounding within the body at the same time. This deeper opening gradually occurs and is greatly helped by the upward assimilation of sexual energy. These nectars keep our cosmic energy in the body from being too fiery and mental by invoking the watery and fluidic aspects.

There are times when your crown opens up so much that you expand tremendously and your body feels like the tiniest speck in a large sea of consciousness. Walking around in a body in this state is truly a humbling experience. In this state we firsthand understand the lack of an independent soul, but the sea of bliss more than makes up for the loss of egoic solidity.

There are understandings of our nature and destiny that can only be understood within this experience, however it is a mistake to think that this buddhic experience is the ultimate. It is more like one end of a spectrum, a node of existence if you will. The fuller experience in regards to liberation in form is much more tantric in nature and has this expanded state incorporated within it in an indescribable manner.

One of the primary dangers of drugs such as marijuana is its effect upon the pineal gland, occipitals and temples. Marijuana and similar drugs cause the pineal gland to go out of alignment, often encasing it with a fog and also actually misaligning the etheric energy it receives with its physical point of grounding. This can be disastrous in terms of spiritual discrimination, essentially loosing ones way and increasing delusion. The only positive spiritual effect these drugs have is that they help some people to open their hearts more (thus letting go and letting god as the saying goes), but at a price.

This space in the center of your head is a cave of incredible value. Within this cave an indescribable subtle space can be experienced, resonating with the universe itself, and the blissful joy of feeling this creates nectar in the body. It feels so clear, like space itself, bright, bubbling and knowing.

Lower Back of the Head

The lower back of the head is a storage area for refined sexual juices, which is then fed to your brain and down into your body. The lower back of the head has been called "the mouth of God," both for the subtle nectar that can collect there and for its transparent connection into your environment. In the process of opening it many visions may be seen and loud sounds may be heard.

The nectars in the back of the head can support a bi-local experience. Similar to the way that we have two arms, we can have more than one place where our expression interacts with the environment. Because our two arms are part of our body as a whole, we do not feel that we have one body for one arm and another for the other, even though each arm can be doing a different activity. Similarly, when our identity is consciousness itself, we can have multiple activities.

The exact spot is just above the soft area above the occipital and inwards. When first concentrating in this area, toxins released from the occipital region can make it quite sore. By withdrawing your energy into this chakra, you may feel yourself entering a subtle sphere of existence and the ability to inwardly view other places. Through continued concentration this area is sometimes felt as an eye in the back of your head and the back of your body feels just like your front.

The back of the head directly supports your third eye through an energy conduit that passes through the center of the head. As such,

Kriya yogis often focus on first opening the back of the head before focusing through the third eye. The Kriya Yogis draw upon nectars from the back of the head to nourish the body and support a refined consciousness. This is done through a combination of visualization, directed breath and sometimes seductively stimulating the back of the upper palette with the tongue.

Focussing in the back of your head may make you feel a little spacey and thus is not recommended before going to work in the morning or before driving a car.

Soma Point (upper back of head)

This small chakra is located in the upper back of the head, about 1/3 of the way down from top of the head to the occipitals. You can receive nourishment by visualizing white star-light enter this area and condense into a substance that is collected at the lower back of the head and the throat center.

This is a very transcendent activity often overseen by the energy of Shiva. It requires the ability to remain with the subtle stream of nectar sometimes amidst a very eclectic display of activity often thrashing with fifth dimensional beings of distortion and power-hunger and thus is not for the socially bound, ambitiously driven or meek-hearted personality.

When Mahavatar BabaJi showed me this technique he had me visualize that I was sitting on the dark side of the moon while doing this. For myself, the starlight that came in through the head was felt to originate from and as Mahavatar BabaJi.

The soma point has a pure and somewhat direct connection into the central channel and thus is a place that can both stimulate and assimilate desire.

I have witnessed that some of the Tibetan Powa masters, in transferring the essence of others and in part their own consciousness into higher realms, are in fact moving into a higher astral realm connected with this soma point, while other Tibetan Masters are moving into the higher realms directly through the crown of the head. As to the opening directly above the head, I can fully follow, while as to the transference through the soma point, I can only partially follow, but feel that this is not the fullness of the enlightened abodes of the ascended masters/deities, rather a temporary playground. However, there may be further activity on those realms entered by the soma point I have not witnessed, so this is only an incomplete observation.

Forehead (third eye)

The third eye refers to a point of focus and an inner-space between the two eyebrows (and often a little upwards). The third eye has a cooling nature to it that is strengthening and calming to the body.

As with all the chakras, different colors may be emphasized at different times. Colors often used in conjunction with concentrating or generating prana at the third eye include white, blue, violet, gold, pink and red. For example, red for energizing, blue for its natural deep quality, pink for softening, white for strengthening, violet for energizing, purifying and deepening, gold for projecting, etc.

The actual focal point of the third eye may change from the bridge of the nose, up to between the eyebrows and up the forehead several inches. The lower part is more connected to your body and the upper reaches is transcendent and free of the body. This change in focus results from where you are collecting the nectars along this part of the central channel and is effected by the details of your focus within your body and environment. Start by focusing between the eyebrows about an inch or so inwards and slightly upwards and feel a collection of fluidic consciousness supporting a sense that you can see within an inner space. Do not focus hard on seeing, rather just relax in the sense that you can. It is this sense that opens up the inner-space. As you gain this ability, occasionally become aware of a tube about a ¼ inch in diameter in which you are centered. The tube moves up the forehead (and continues to the top of the head and back down the spine). Move up a few inches and then back down, so that you can experience for yourself the different aspects of the third eye. Move slowly, perhaps only an inch at a sitting, so that you bring the actual ecstatic substance through that tube and gain the definition of it.

Focusing at the third eye during still meditation can stimulate energy and thus keep you more awake. However, if the extra energy is not absorbed or circulated, then the stagnation of energy itself will lead to a sleepy and dull state. If you are in a wakeful, yet turbulent way, it is better to focus in the lower body at first. As energy builds in the third eye, learn to "drop it" down into the throat, the heart, and the navel.

The third eye is considered the upper aperture of the central channel running through the center of the body. However, when the central channel is extended through the top of the head, then the opening to the third eye is a branch. It has a connection through polarity with the lower end of the fusion channel at the tip of the penis or vagina. The third eye also has a natural connection with the navel and tan-tien. A practitioner should not try to advance the opening of their third eye ahead of its receiving energetic support from the navel and lower centers. This requires the opening of at least one of the vertical energy channels of the body.

For a person wanting visionary development through the third eye area, it is recommended to develop this in conjunction with the heart chakra. By opening the heart and third-eye together, not rushing ahead in one at the expense of the other, wholeness develops and you will see by feeling and feel as you see. This gives a better grounding and depth of inner sight where everything is felt "as within." This is extremely important, so that a person goes deeper, rather than becomes sidetracked by phenomena.

Feeling allows us to move not just through the three dimensions of inner space, but also through the deepening of inner space itself, because we can feel ourselves deeper and gain the instantaneous feedback of knowingness. The opening of the third eye and heart together is an aspect of the central channel called the amrita nadi, which is buddhic consciousness.

The third eye is a common point of focus for many yogic practices. With practice, it is an easy chakra to hold a focus at. There are a number of energy channels all in close proximity to each other at the third eye, and this makes it easier to bring everything together in a central focus.

The third eye is commonly associated with mental focus and the ability to control the mind and its direction. It is not that a yogi tries to control every thought. Rather when the prana is purified sufficiently and brought deep enough so that it enters the central channel the thoughtless and alert state is naturally experienced.

I recommend that a beginning practitioner spend a moderate amount of time focusing on the third eye; that is not too much. It is much more important at this stage to strengthen the general grounding in the body and opening of the flows of energy that support a wholesome feeling. Too much initial focus in the head can create heat and a heady feeling that is not at all desirable.

As the channels in the head and the body as a whole become open there will be no heady feeling whatsoever by focusing at the third eye or within any of the other head centers. The third eye area can hold and focus regenerating nectars for the body.

As the third eye opens in conjunction with the other chakras in the head, it creates a very expansive feeling and vision. Fine nectars collect around the third eye that can best be described as a refinement of the sexual juices, like the sweet and ecstatic nectar experienced in a woman's vagina during lovemaking. It gives a wonderful quality to the personality and presence. This is an important part of creating the tantric or rejuvenating body. As it is first tasted at the third eye, the feeling of this nectar is then used for further development of the third eye. Preceding this awareness, a filling out of energy gradually occurs as the sexual energy is brought upwards and blended in each area of the body. This nectar prana can qualify the intake of prana from above the head into more nectar and also gives the substance to develop a fine body, which can travel in the subtle realms. This same process can also be done in other chakras.

Collecting, refining, and generating this nectar at the third eye is the best way of fully developing its potential. Within this field of nectar you can develop a subtle body. You should physically feel the area of the third eye and clear the channels that go to each side, the channel that goes back into the center of the head, and the forward projection into space. Opening the third eye in this way strengthens the whole body as well.

Arc-Line

The arc-line is a term presented by Yogi Bhajan corresponding to the upper forehead. It has an outward nature, and thus is a natural pranic support for presence and projection. When your arc-line is activated, you can see your own radiant image; at first your head and at times your entire body. This is not an imagination, but an actual, radiant, very bright vision that occurs spontaneously when this faculty is developed.

There are several energetic supports which all come together to create a strong arc-line. There is vital substance from the body which is brought up and distilled from the lower body into the back of the head and forehead. The nectar at the third eye then spreads across the forehead to the temples. Finally, and perhaps the most important, your presence from directly above the head, what I call the eighth chakra flows down into the pineal gland and then through the third eye and forehead region and mixes with the nectars in the head to create a confident fullness across the entire forehead and within the temples as well.

There is an intimate connection with the temples and the kidneys. First focus at the third eye and then spread out this presence to the temples. Next energetically connect the temples to your kidneys. In this way you can "hold" a space in which to heal and fill out your kidneys using breath, feeling and visualization. By holding a supportive space from the arc-line you can overcome subtle obstructions and blocks that might otherwise make this more difficult.

Chakras above the Head

Only a brief mention will be made here as this is the subject of Eternal Yoga (the next book in this series).

It is only appropriate to **attempt to fully** enter into this area **after** a spiritual foundation has been created, including purification, fulfillment, integration and maturing of experience. Otherwise, as we have seen many times, projection into these spheres of activity simply becomes delusion and distraction. The mind can and does create its own reality, and this reality can become a spiritual trap, reinforced by others of like-mind. Rather than transcend one's particular bindings, this can reinforce them, by bringing one right into the seed energy, yet without a way to recognize it as other than that. For example subtle collective karmas that we are a part of. There is a danger of subtle pride that can carry on for many lifetimes. These realms only become safely workable from a viewpoint beyond mind.

While there are a number of chakras near the outside of the head, the eighth chakra is of principle interest. This chakra contains the blueprint for the bodily chakra system. It is used in a generic fashion through visualizations of light and presence entering from above the head into the body, such as visualizing ones teacher or guides above the head. This is a good way to start and may be safely used. Next there is a chakra about 3 to 6 feet above the head that is of a very expanded and subtle mental essence. Moving up an octave, we go to a chakra far above the head. The spatial distance is an effective physiological way of relating this energy into normal consciousness. This chakra is a gateway to realms beyond the light. Within this are two more chakras corresponding to a higher octave of the eighth and ninth center.

This corresponds to a total of 12 chakras/realms. There is no such thing as the 13th or 14th chakra etc., however there are infinite ways that consciousness can relate within these realms, yet consciousness itself experienced in this way is unchanging.

The distance above the head is purely a practical relationship. In reality, these realms are beyond this kind of spatial representation. For example, they may be entered through a chakra within the physical body.

CHANNELS

Our body is made of energy, and within this maze of energy are concentrated flows. As an analogy compare cells and energy. Our entire body consists of cells and a number of these cells are blood. Some types of cells stay put and some types of cells move around fluidly connecting everything together (blood for example). Within this sea of blood lie major flows of it known as arteries. Similarly, there are major conduits or flows of energy (prana) in our body which we may call channels (channels of energy or nadis).

While we can see blood, most of us cannot see energy, only its effects such as being alive, having enough energy, feeling great, etc. Yet, with practice we can learn to directly perceive, feel, and eventually gain direct identity with energy as an aspect of consciousness itself.

All of the energy routes presented in this chapter are inside the physical body. While there are auric projections of these flows or parts of these flows that extend beyond the body, for the most part, it is better to visualize, connect with, and energize these flows from within the physical body. That is not to say that all of these energy channels exist in the physical, just that there spatial reference in relation to the physical is within (or should be within) the physical body.

Just as arteries can become clogged and less fit to support life, so can our energy channels become clogged and blocked. A lot of the preliminary work of clearing these energy flows can be done through the dynamic yoga sets given in this book. Visualization combined with breathing is an excellent way to get more familiar with your flows of energy and to further clear and vitalize them.

By becoming familiar with our energy channels, we start to awaken within our energy body, thus expanding our range of awareness and interaction. Just as a baby learns to ground within its new body, exploring it, finding its boundaries and being in it, correspondingly the process of grounding within our energy body brings us a new body of awareness.

While there are many flows of energy in the body, the principle routes are those connected with our chakras. The chakras exist within these flows, and the flows unite the chakras as one big energy mass. In this book we will explore the principal vertical channels, which are the microcosmic orbit and the central channel, as well as briefly touching in on some of the horizontal flows, such as the belt channel at the navel. In a sense the chakras are also horizontal flows as they create a horizontal wheel of activity around them.

There are many other flows of energy, such as the acupuncture meridians within the organs and tissues of the body. These flows are connected to the deeper underlying principal flows previously mentioned. While of much value, the acupuncture meridians are not directly discussed in this book (except for the spinal, frontal, and fusion (central) meridians. Simply, we start somewhere and from that starting point eventually the whole picture is embraced, then it does not matter what name we call an energy, or where we reference it, it is the spiritual blissful-wholeness that counts. When happiness wells within us, we just feel happy, similarly when the spiritual bliss of our being takes hold, it is the spirit that is acknowledged. Thus the channels, chakras, essences, and energy awaken to become our body of bliss and it is our spirit that is acknowledged.

While at first it is helpful and conducive to think of the principal energy flows like rivers, in advanced stages of practice this can interfere with a proper understanding. As you advance, these flows actually contain phenomenal amounts of potential-energy-substance and in this way they are more like lakes or oceans with a current running through a part of them, like an undersea ocean current. This current is what is referred to as "the flow or channel," but in reality is only the part you have actualized. By only focusing on this "flow," you may be keeping your mind on its outer aspect and miss the ocean. This ocean is your spiritual body, and the minuscule part of it we call the channels are what you are relating to. In the beginning it is better and more effective to simply think of the channels like rivers within your body and learn to generate and be aware of the current. In advanced stages of practice, however the situation reverses and your physical body is generated from an effortless current within this cosmic ocean of your being. This might be misinterpreted to indicate that you should focus on the channels as being physically larger and larger in size, but this is a misunderstanding of the inner nature. It is better to keep the channels in a small size in relation to the body, and the inner-expanse will fill out. This can only be understood in a non-dual awareness.

Microcosmic Orbit

The microcosmic orbit is the first energy flow you should become familiar with. It travels along the spine into the head, continuing to the crown, the third eye and the down the front, underneath, and then continues up the spine. Energy can and does travel in both directions, although for most people and most of the time, down the front and up the back is the normal and recommended direction to focus upon. When your tongue touches the upper roof of the mouth this connects the flow from the third eye down the front of your body. Opening up the perineum and tailbone area connects the frontal flow through the perineum and up the back.

The microcosmic orbit, as are all the energy flows of the body, is originally parented by the portion of the central channel directly above the head, and then through the central channel within the body. For most practitioners this is simply esoteric knowledge, but as you continue to develop in your practice and experience your body emanating out of your central core, then it becomes practical.

Usually, it is best to start with the frontal aspect. The frontal line is your emotional presence and projection and thus is intimately connected with the organs of your body. Because of this emotional vitality, the frontal line becomes the first receptacle of your breath. As you inhale, breathe down the frontal line to the tan-tien and exhale while keeping the subtle energy of your breath at the tan-tien or another area below the solar plexus. As you build some energy in the frontal line then as you inhale bring it to the perineum (about an inch or so before the anus) and as you exhale, bring it up the spine and all the way to the third eye.

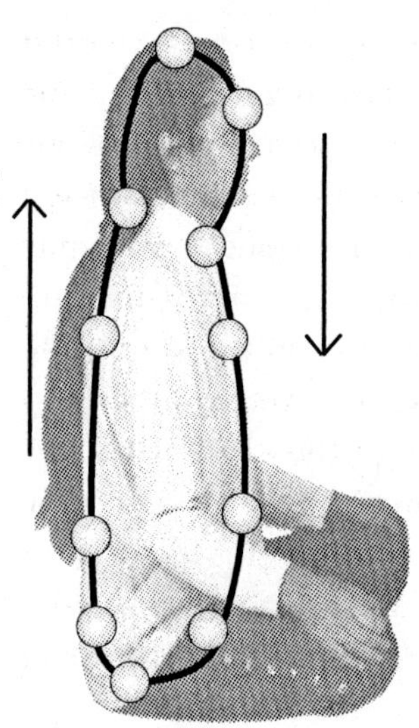

At first you may find it more effective to break up the orbit into two cycles of the breath. Inhale down to the tan-tien, exhale to the perineum or to the tailbone. Inhale to the large bone at the back of the neck and exhale to the third eye for one complete circuit.

After you experience at least a subtle sense of energy in the orbit as you circulate through it with your mind, you may want to ignore having to do the whole orbit on only one or two rounds of the breath. Instead, move the energy around a small amount on the exhale, then keep track of where it is while inhaling. Then on the exhale move the energy a little bit more on the circuit. This helps you to really feel what you are doing, and you can spend time getting an energy awareness focused through areas you have difficulty with.

Another approach is to breath slowly and deeply, but to ignore having to link the breath and the mind together through an in and out movement. Rather the breath helps to create a potent sea of energy available for the mind to draw on continually as you explore and move through the orbit. But for all these variations, you should first practice for awhile with a normal linking of the breath to movement through the orbit taking one or two breaths to complete the cycle. Even if in the beginning you think it is all your imagination, you are in fact gradually increasing the vitality of the channel, developing a better whole body sense, and learning how to connect the mind to the body and breath.

After you have gained connectivity to the orbit, most often the next step is to pick an area to build energy, which you will then use to circulate through the orbit. At this stage it is also good to be able to differentiate the difference between the surface of the spine and deep within the marrow. Practice circulating energy both ways and feel the difference for yourself. This will be discussed in more depth latter in this chapter.

You may read that it is dangerous to open the microcosmic orbit. Perhaps if you are going about this is the traditional way, sealing yourself in a room or cave for 49 days and meditating for 3 or 4 sessions, each of several hours per day, and you force the energy through a wrong path or build up too much energy in an organ you may create a serious upset to the body. But be serious, most people are starting with a much more mundane practice and in the beginning cannot direct enough energy to hurt themselves even if they tried on purpose. Apply common sense, do not over force anything, ask for help if you have a question, listen to your body, and do not be fanatical, and you will be fine.

The prime symptom to watch out for is congestion of energy in one area. You may notice this as soreness, bloating, pain or just uncomfortableness. This can happen because there is blockage that does not allow the energy to flow through that point. It can also occur through a weakening that disperses the energy to the surrounding tissues where it build up. In this case, back to listening to your body. Persist only for a reasonable time, then do something else to move the energy. Go for a walk, massage the area and the body, relax.

Some detoxification is normal and small amounts of discomfort are acceptable. But do not rush the whole process too quickly. If in doubt ask for help. Particularly as the lower torso become tonified, you may experience some bloating and gas. This will pass.

When you are ready to pick a place to build large amounts of energy to use for the orbit, listed below are some options. The safest to use and recommended for most people is the lower tan-tien, which is just below the navel. The other options are available for experienced practitioners, although often then navel area is still the best place to start.

- Through gentle and consistent mediation building your presence at the third eye, which is a miniature you. This has a lot of intelligence and innate radiance in it, thus as you gradually circulate this down the front, it (you) know how to gather, refine and blend energy along the way. When it reaches down to the solar plexus and tan-tien area it further blends itself with the emotional strength of this area, which gives it greater form and integration into the wholeness of who you are. This creates a lot of energy, which continues in the orbit, circulating up the spine and around and around. The advantage of this approach if done correctly, is that it can directly transform the mental energy in your head to a nectar feeling, thus overcoming at the start a potential limitation of directing energy through the body with the mind (that of inherent separation between your mental thought and the actual energy itself desired to be moved).

  There are a number of fine points to successfully using the energy of the third eye to fully open up the microcosmic orbit. The first is to sufficiently develop the nectar at the third eye, and this can take a few years. The next is to develop a strong sense that you can see the entire body from within the third eye. With this ability you can then awaken all the chakras and the energy route through an inner activation from the third eye. It is as if all the chakras exist in the third eye itself, which from the subtle realms is a reality. However, this is far beyond mere imagination, for when you see a chakra or energy pathway form the third eye, your energy is also solidity present in actuality at that point or within that flow. This is an approach used within the kriya path.

- Breathing and visualizing energy in the frontal area of the solar plexus or tan-tien, cultivating a moist fire and magnetic attraction of energy in this area, often as a golden-white substance. As this builds, there is lots of vitality to circulate in the orbit. This works particularly well with breathing exercises and is perhaps the most commonly recommended start. One must be careful to internalize the energy and surrender it into the empty-radiance of enlightenment. The advantage of this approach is that the energy starts less mental and more vital than other approaches. For further tips, read the chapter 12: "an introduction to a tantra of inner fire."

- Connecting with your presence and image above the head, which enters into your body and moves down the frontal line, activating all the energy of your body to resonate with its youthful fire. This continues around the orbit, clearing and energizing it. The advantage of this approach is that it directly originates from a deeper level of your being.

This can be used as a supplemental technique to the others, particularly to get you in touch with the seed karmas behind a blockage that you are having trouble clearing. It is also helpful to bring in the energy of a master.

To fully apply this technique as the energy source to open the microcosmic orbit, you should already be awake in the budhic realms and understand the subtle traps you can create for yourself there. You should also understand the difference between the central channel and the microcosmic orbit. Normally energy from above the head is first brought down into the body through the central channel. This is all discussed in detail in the next book of this series, "Eternal Yoga, Awakening within Budhic Awareness" (see appendix).

The spinal energy is a masculine quality that gives a transcendent and expansively penetrating exactness. Within yogic practice the innermost reaches of the major chakras are often first connected to within the spinal marrow, with the frontal line being part of their projection and energetic play. Later on, as the frontal and spinal energy is mixed back into its source within the central channel, the heart of these chakras then shifts into this central flow. However, it is recommended for practical reasons that you first learn and emphasize the microcosmic orbit.

In the beginning this circulation of energy simply feels like our imagination. Take it slowly and let the mind sink into where it is placed. Breathe vitality into the area of your focus, so that you can feel the response.

If you cannot connect to a part of the flow, then after persevering for five or ten minutes, stop the full cycle and instead inhale and exhale energy through that particular region as a way to build presence and awareness there. When you start to feel something then slowly, move a feeling of energy through that part of the orbit. Finish with the complete orbit and then bring everything into the navel area for a few moments with a contained feeling. By placing the mind slightly in front of an energy mass, you can help move it to its next place, and so on.

It is highly recommended that you learn to work with this flow. It is practical and tremendously beneficial whatever your desire - from enjoying a better life, to spiritual development and definition. Connectivity with this flow is a natural development within a grounded spiritual path and a recommended prerequisite for more advanced practices. Opening this pathway gives you more energy, sensitivity, wholeness, and allows you to balance or integrate the effects of your practices much more easily.

The ability to quickly balance energy in the microcosmic orbit becomes very valuable in intermediate level practices, because if you cause energy to become congested in an area, you have the means to remove that congestion. The ability to quickly balance your energy also keeps a correct perspective of integration and freshness, as well as endurance for longer sittings. Practicing the microcosmic flow clears blockages both in your body and the effects those blockages have on your outlook, essentially you feel able and willing to live life in your chosen direction.

In the beginning visualize the orbit open and easy. Do not be too technical. That is, guide your presence in the whole circuit without letting there be blockages. If there are blockages, then relax into a sense that you move through them anyway. If still you are not doing it, then relax the mind and just make it go in the circle. While at first it is not likely to be that connected or powerful, practice it for at least a few minutes anyway, because it will have some effect, and it is after all, the whole orbit you are opening.

After comprehending the basic circulatory path of energy, the next step is to refine your connectivity to it, bring more energy through it, and clear blockages to that energy on all levels. Most of your work in opening this circuit occurs through combining your breath and mind together. If you do not understand how to feel the subtle current of the breath, then do some of the breathing techniques in this book to develop that ability. Also make sure that the orbit is inside the body, not outside of it.

When you can feel a greater balance and refreshment from circulating your energy through the microcosmic orbit it is time to start working with the specifics. The feeling of refreshment is a key. As feeling-vitality is increased this practice is not a chore, rather a fun activity, like making love, or doing something you enjoy. It is full of surprises, openings, new feelings, tingles, seductive sensations, strength, challenges...

After this initial introduction, to really open up the microcosmic orbit, you need to create an energy source to pump through this orbit. This is usually done at the lower abdomen, or one of the options detailed earlier. This energy is guided through the various places along the orbit. You might emphasize each place for a few days, weeks, or months during your practice, before continuing to the next. In the course of doing this, you will connect with the organs and chakras of each of those places.

Dynamic yoga sets and kriyas clear blockages, create vitality, circulate energy, and bring connectivity of mind, body, energy and movement. Thus these practices are a natural support for the specific focus of opening this orbit to a greater capacity.

Extending the Microcosmic Orbit through the Legs and Outside of the Body

Since the microcosmic orbit is used to gain definition and a sense of wholeness, it becomes natural to extend the scope of this orbit. This expansion is first done by combining the legs as part of the orbit. Energy is brought down your front to the perineum, then down the back of the legs to the feet, then up the front of the legs to the perineum, up the spine and so forth. Thus there will be a figure eight with the crossing point at the perineum. Later (not too soon, so as to keep enough potency of containment), energy can be split at the back of the heart and also circulated through the arms. Further extensions of the orbit can be done by imagining a replication of your body beneath your feet and above the head and continuing the orbit through the pathways of each of theses imaginary bodies. Before this extension above the head is done in earnest, I believe it is better and more beneficial to do the initiatory meditations of Eternal Yoga (as given in the next book in this series) and begin opening the central (fusion) channel. Do these extensions of your bodily awareness first through the fusion channel because it is more connected to the heart of your essence as an alive being.

The microcosmic orbit is also called the small circulation (or small universe) in martial arts and Taoist practices (I learned it through the internal marital arts). As it is extended into the arms, legs, all the meridians and into cosmic circulations of energy it is called the large orbit. Generally, the small orbit is filled out first, before the large orbit is begun. Otherwise there is not enough internal energy available for the circulation, and also focusing on the large orbit first tends to make the energy external and thus not internal, thus interfering with the meditative deepening and strengthening of bodily and spiritual awareness.

When the large orbit is begun, there are many methods. One approach is to start by generating a lot of energy in the arms or legs and pulling it in to connect with the already internalized energy. Another is to visualize the internalized energy expanding out through the arms and legs. Commonly, a combination of the two approaches is used. The general visualization of the arms and legs as a whole are safe, however specific and repeated visualizations through the circuit of the meridians as outlined in some books must be overseen by a person who has already mastered this, so that serious upsets in the bodies energy are not created.

The large orbit also includes establishing a greater connectivity and integrity of the small orbit to the organs and tissues of the body. There are many ways of doing this. I feel one of the best is through a combination with organ, tissues and bone breathing as introduced in chapter seven: "The Magic of Breathing."

While someone interested in the martial arts will expand the small circulation into the large circulation through the arms and legs, a person more interested in the spiritual benefits will probably move from the small circulation into the central (fusion) channel and then into cosmic aspects of the body. In this case, expansion into the arms and legs simply through yoga sets and simply chi kung is sufficient. Also you may want to incorporate five-gates breathing, which is sitting, being relaxed and opening the palms of the hands, soles of the foot and top of the head. Then a subtle breath is felt through these five points connecting to the inner landscape of your body, often coordinated by awareness at the third eye and tan-tien.

I would like to address a criticism made by a few Taoist practitioners regarding other yogic practices, such as Kundalini yoga and how they do not mix cooling earth energy or ground enough into the body, i.e., overheating the head. This may happen due to incorrect practice, imbalance of the masculine and feminine nature, keeping energy on the outer aspects, ignorance, or immaturity in practice. This commonly happens when technicians without inner mastery teach these techniques. It then becomes a hit or miss affair. While some yogic paths do not describe the microcosmic orbit specifically they do circulate energy through various combinations of channels, passions, transmission, and a natural quality of opening. When these techniques are matured, the energy deepens into the central channel, which is the melding place of all technique and all paths of wholesomeness. Another point to remember is that the outer kriyas are not meant to be a path complete in itself, just as the microcosmic orbit is not a complete spiritual path in itself. They serve a valuable function to prepare the way for more internal meditations, such as the inner tantras.

The Side Channels

Every principal vertical energy flow in the body, such as the frontal line, the spine, and the central channel each has one or more pairs of supporting flows of energy that accompany it. Each of these pairs consists of a more masculine and a more feminine channel. What follows is a discussion of the side channels that accompany the central and spinal channels. The term "side" indicates that the channels are primarily located to the left and right side of the primary channel they accompany, in comparison to the front and back for example.

Before we embark into a greater understanding of the side channels, it is important to understand the perspective in which we will be applying this knowledge.

The key to tantric embodiment is learning how to ground within our central channel. The central channel, which is discussed in greater detail elsewhere in this chapter, is our spiritual core out of which we experience our body and world. More than an actual location it is a state of non-dual consciousness, but for practical purposes that become evident as we continue on a tantric path, it is important to define its location as a channel of energy and abode of consciousness in relation to our body. Thus one of the principle reasons of using the side channels is to make firm the central channel. To return to this primal experience we dissolve our pranas and thus consciousness back into this core, and to achieve liberation we learn how to consciously and simultaneously emanate out of and dissolve into this core in a dynamic uncontrived balance, which is another way of saying that we are totally one-hundred percent physically integrated with the natural state. Spiritually, the reason for foundational practices such as presented in this book is to gradually increase our ability to apply ourselves in this way.

As the central channel in essence is emptiness, until this becomes totally integrated with everyday experience, the inner qualities of the central channel lie beyond our experience of physicality. As a bridge to localizing this core within our being, it is common to start with the spine and more particularly the spinal marrow. The back of the spine, close to and along the skin is more of a fiery somewhat mental quality. The marrow is more of a watery, sensational quality. Because this quality of the spinal marrow is deep, this helps us to connect with our central channel, and thus the terms spinal (marrow) channel and central channel our often used interchangeably, although technically they are not the same thing. For example some practitioners find it more helpful to visualize the central channel in front of the spinal marrow.

This inflowing and out flowing of prana from the central and spinal channels most strongly occurs through their accompanying side channels. Our sexual essence of blood and semen are nectars that support these pranas and thus bringing the refined essence of our blood and semen into the side channels gives a tremendous support to this prana. This also allows these essences to better enter the central channel itself and thereby act as an integrative force, i.e., a bridge between our blissful formless consciousness and bodily identity. Even if we do not differentiate the energy of our side channels into masculine and feminine qualities, just directing our prana into them will greatly help to firm the central channel. For some this is enough. You must experiment for yourself, observer yourself and see what works. Must of us need some help along the way. There is no one fixed formula. If you want to progress on the tantric path - then really get this, otherwise everything gets stuck. Yes there is a science, but there is also an art. This is one of the reasons why we need a teacher, for a teacher understands the art.

In general, internal, receptive and nurturing qualities are dominant on the left side of our body and active, outgoing qualities on the right. For example, many people are more sensitive to taking in and feeling another person on their left side than on their right. Thus it is natural to relate the right side of our body with a masculine identity and the left side of the body with a feminine identity.

In general yogic disciplines we use this understanding of the left and right side of the body accordingly. For example, in a twisting exercise, we breathe in as we twist to the left as the left side is our receiving side (in-breath) and we breathe out as we twist to the right. Another example is if our right side is contracting, then we might look at masculine issues, for example, are we outward enough. However in tantric yoga as we ground deeper within our channels, this convenient and clear-cut definition of the two sides of the body falls away, as will be explained.

For men, much of the prana to give strength and clarity comes from their semen, and thus cultivation and refinement of semen greatly supports a man on the spiritual path. Yet semen itself, white in color, is earthy, moon-like and cool in essence. While aggressive outward activity helps to create energy for the production of semen, semen itself is lunar in essence, a feminine quality. While a man has a strong mental body, it is the seminal fluids more than any other substance that allows the grounding of this into the body. Because of this earthy feminine like quality of semen, when it is clarified within the channels it tends to flow more on the left side of the spine.

While women have a seminal like fluid produced sexually, the support of feminine qualities is contained more in the blood and the organs. Feminine blood, which of course is larger in volume than semen and present in every cell of the body, is more naturally richer in certain qualities than for a man. One of the qualities of blood is energy and heat. Thus while the feminine qualities are soft and passive, which allows for nourishment, the actual quality of blood is energetic and expansive. Thus it is natural for the essence energy of blood (not the blood itself) to flow through the channels of the right side of the body more than the left.

Thus what results is that for men, whose outward character is more on the right side of the body, are inwardly better contained on the left side channel, and visa versa for women. This is the exact opposite of our outward bodily characteristics. This is a tremendously valuable understanding in teaching us how to work with, contain and expand our energy tantrically through the inner channels.

Before we get too set in this formula, understand that it changes again and again, i.e., what was previously identified as masculine becomes seen in a feminine light, and visa versa. Also in a sense all our bodily energies are feminine in nature with the masculine polarity being the formless, and even this in a certain light changes. But for the purpose of collecting our sexual essences and prana into the side channels, the previously mentioned and practical understanding is adequate.

This natural switching of masculine energy to the left and feminine to the right has many benefits. This changing of polarities is one example of what Taoist terminology calls "threading the energy." One of the benefits is that there is a preliminary blending, i.e., the masculine and feminine energies on the right side and the masculine and feminine energies on the left side. This results through the polarity of attraction an energetic increase, elevation and containment of energy in each of the side channels. This deepening makes it easier for the energy to more naturally enter into the central channel. It is important that the correct depth of the central channel is entered, i.e., entering into the actual central channel that is characteristic of our spirit, rather than just the body's outer physiology. This preliminary blending helps the energy of the left and right channels to come closer to the spinal marrow and central channel which thereby firms the location of the central channel and increases the bliss felt within it. Another benefit is that the masculine strength becomes experienced not so much as outer activity but as an inner stillness. For woman, there is experienced much more of an energetic empowerment which can overcome passive tendencies on the spiritual path.

Now that we have covered the perspective in which the side channels are used, i.e., to firm and support the central channel, along with an understanding of how we can tantrically qualify the energies within the side channels, let us review their pathways in the body.

To understand the shape and pathways a flow of energy takes in our bodies, we must understand that these flows can be experienced and described either independent of the body, i.e., in an inner space, or else in direct and exact relationship with the body, for example corresponding with a sensation through a path of muscles, blood, nerves, etc. Yet even when we describe these essential energy flows in direct relation to the body, this can change if we change the nature of the energy flow itself. For example, a flow of energy can move more towards the surface of the body or deeper within it, and it can change its apparent pathway through the body altogether. The same energy can occur simultaneously through several paths at once. What this ultimately leads up to is that our whole body is simply one energy flow, or in a better light, a sea of currents. But for practical application, it is better to create more definition and separation, so we will give different names to the different pathways that a particular flow can travel.

Except as stated in the following paragraphs, we should visualize and feel the side channels close to the primary channel. Initially, the best way to feel these channels is through their stimulation of the muscles running along side the spine, often felt as a pleasant current, perhaps warmth and a tingling of sensation. It is suggested to start connecting to the side channels about an inch to and inch and a half to each side of the spine, running straight. However, it is common for beginners that the energy loops out into space in certain places, or else we find it running much further away from the spine. Keep practicing and persisting at bringing it closer in, not outside of the body. There are a set of meridians that run several inches out to each side of the spine that are necessary for the support of more grosser emotions and organ vitality. Until we refine ourselves, the energy may want to find its way to this outer flow, but if you stay at it and honestly and with spiritual depth work through any emotions that come up, the energy will move inwards. There is also a line of energy that runs along the side of our body. Splitting some of our awareness to flow down the sides of our body for a few minutes can help to create more bodily prana and general containment.

In terms of a color, make the left side, our seminal and seminal like essence, white. Make our blood like essence on the right side red. Sometimes you use color and sometimes it is best to forget about it. As a further distinction, you can visualize the channels (energy flows) as flexible semitransparent tubes containing energy substance. This is purely a guide and not an absolute correspondence to the way it is, however it can be extremely helpful in containing our energy so that it build the necessary potency and being able to control and guide it in relation to our body. In spiritual application, a practical visualization even if is not absolute truth is often more effective, for it helps us gain connectivity and a taste. Without connectivity there is neither potency nor integration and nothing advances at all.

In regards to the side channels, the primary distinction is focusing on them as running straight besides or else intertwining around the spinal or central channel. After this primary distinction there are flows that run closer to the spine and farther out from it. Finally, there are applications where parts of the pathway runs straight and some circle around the primary channel at particular chakras (abodes). There are also refinements in paying attention to the myriad branches of the side channels, i.e., connections, throughout the body. Sometimes this is a distraction and other times it is greater integration. In the beginning just keep them straight and close in towards the spinal marrow, i.e., an inch or so under the skin.

The side channels start at each nostril, comes closer to the primary channel at the third eye, then ascends towards the crown and descends down alongside the spinal or central channel to its lower tip. There are various branches, but we will not discuss them at this time. Inside the head the distance from the primary channel is generally a little looser, corresponding to the rich myriad of flows and functions occurring within the head. An important exception is in the area of the third eye, where the proximity of the side channels to the central channel can be used to create rich nectar at the third eye supporting a much higher level of vision.

As the channels approach the lower back of the head, they all come closer together and travel parallel down to near the tip of the spine. A mental energy follows more of a straight line, while a feeling energy follows more of a curvature or spiraling flow. Thus when using more of a mental quality the side channels are felt to run straight. This can allow a direct connection to a subtle place of mind and a mental penetrative quality. It also makes everything simple, and this simplicity helps some to better focus on the central channel, not putting too much acrobatics into the side channels.

However this straightness does not facilitate connectivity to our bodily condition, nor does it best use the energy of our emotions and passions. By intertwining the side channels around the spine, this creates more sensation, which can open up profound inner spaces. When the channels are intertwined with each other, this changes the energy more from a fire or wind quality to a water quality, which thereby brings the energy into a great relationship with the central (fusion) channel. For example, sexual orgasm as most people experience it is generated through energy and fluids moving along the inner set of twirling side channels around the fusion channel. In many of the Tibetan Buddhist tantras, the energy is revolved once around the navel chakra, three times around the heart chakra, once around the throat chakra and once around the crown center. The side energy flows are joined at the third eye and most commonly at the navel chakra (a few inches below the level of the navel point), although sometimes they are joined lower. The rest of the path is straight. This has an advantage of helping to loosen constrictions around each of these chakras and develop a better absorption of energy into and flow out of these centers, essentially opening them up.

An alternative is what Tara showed to me in a dream, where the two side channels intertwine in a tight helix, crossing about every inch and a half.

Finally there is a variation of this continual helix whereby the diameter is about three to six inches and there are of course less crossings. This helix is the outer shell of the central channel also called the fusion channel. It is felt as your masculine and feminine essences making love to each and thus blissful. It helps to make the transition from the spinal marrow to the true central channel. It is very balancing and is much easier to sense that the close in flows, because of its emotional integration and connectivity with the organ. It opens up the inner space and gives an initial understanding of the central channel and emptiness. However, to develop into a more profound entering of the central channel, as well as penetration into our essences, then you should move back into the close in set of energy flows.

Commonly the energies are absorbed into the primary channel at a certain place or places, such as the base of the spine, the navel chakra or third eye for example. This energy once it is absorbed and stilled (deeply felt) is often then further circulated in the primary channel and sometimes re-emitted back out through the side channels and then the body as a whole. The energy can also be re-emitted through a chakra and along its corresponding energy flows that may or may not include the side channels.

There are a number of ways we guide energy into the side channels but generally we use a combination of breath, visualization and connectivity. There are a number of kriyas, some of which are given in this book, whereby we breathe energy in through the nose and either down one side at a time or down both sides simultaneously. Often on the exhale the energy is brought into and up the primary channel. It is important that the center of the breath is kept low in the belly so that we are extracting and guiding the energy aspect of the breath, rather than just its physical air component. Visualization can be used with or without the breath, and it is important that we move slowly in our visualization so that we develop connectivity with energy itself. An example of connectivity, is simply being aware of energy absorbing form all over the body and various organs directly into the side channels. In this was we can then learn how to increase, collect, contain and refine energy as actual tangible substance.

It is possible when intensely focusing on the side channels that you can throw your body out of balance. Taken to an extreme, you may experience excess heat or cold, anger, inconsideration of others, over concern with everyone, delusions, discomfort, hyper sensitivity and diseases which are hard to correct. Once everything is clear and aligned then this can only happen if you intentionally try to make it happen, and why would you want to do that? Previous to this, take your time and ask for help. Primarily, listen to your body. Also always, always do the side channel meditations as a way of entering the central channel, otherwise, you will definitely increase imbalance in the body over time, because you are increasing the pranas that outwardly support our various delusions, rather than seeing through them from a deeper perspective and grounding, which is a gift of the central channel. Ask a teacher for help.

Belt Channel

The belt channel is a rich presence of energy around the waist. This channel is near the skin with connections to the tan-tien (several inches below the navel) and kidneys. This disc of energy also projects out several feet from the body. After you become familiar with the microcosmic orbit, this is the next recommended energy flow to add to your energy awareness.

The belt channel helps to integrate the two sides of the body and through this alignment it helps to integrate your divine image into the world. It makes your kidneys area feel comfortable and strong. By activating awareness of this energy flow, it becomes easier to ground higher energy into the body and thereby feel your own image (within the sea of infinite potential and many images). The internal martial arts emphasize development of the belt channel.

Vitalizing the belt channel helps to gain firm placement of attention within that part of the body and thus is a preliminary to more accurately creating the inner temple and in blending energy through the navel area. Vitalizing the belt channel assists in mixing prana from above and below within the navel chakra. This channel will help you to absorb subtle universal energy and maintain a positive attitude. This positively is particularly potent when the belt channel helps to maintain alignment of the pineal gland within your body. You can touch in with this feeling by doing the eternal yoga meditation of connecting with your presence above the head (particularly a few inches to six feet up) and then simultaneously becoming aware of the belt channel and its projected energy disc.

For a general start, rather than circulate energy in a loop in this channel, I feel it is better to simply feel it full all at once. Start either in the front and go around both sides to the back, or start in the back and go around both sides to the front, then simply feel a potency and energy in the entire area. There may be some rumblings in your intestines, and balancing of energy. Remember that the belt channel is not an end to itself, but an energetic support that may be used in internalizing energy in the navel or tan-tien chakras and from there into the central channel, or used as an energy source for the microcosmic orbit.

As you connect more with your kidneys, then it is good to feel energy-substance from each kidney flowing an inch or two under the skin around the belt to the tan-tien in the front, about an inch and a half below the navel and a few inches inwards. For example, kidney essence from your left kidney would flow around the left side to the tan tien, and kidney-essence from your right kidney would flow around the right side to the tan-tien. When they meet in the tan-tien, they create a peasant warmth. This is also coordinated with your breath, breathing down into the tan-tien and radiating out from it. As this become full, you may want to direct the energy from the tan-tien inwards towards the spine, and from there it radiates up the spinal marrow and through the body.

Mantak Chia teaches a visualization in his books of spiraling energy from the belt channel up the whole body, simultaneously inside it, on the surface and around it. Your rib cage contains a very creative energy that is stimulated in this way. This spiral also helps to fill out the disk-like energy and integration of the other chakras, and stimulates the very outer aspects of the central channel (also known as the fusion channel).

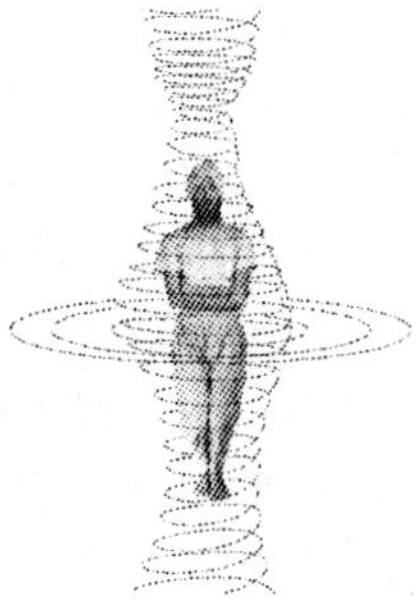

Central Channel

This is your core. It is how your spirit first enters into the body. This could also be called the bliss channel. Connecting with this depth is creating the inner temple. It is the foundation of Tantra and the unification of inner and outer. Shifting primary awareness into the central (fusion) channel is not a beginning step, rather, with some exceptions, one that is usually begun a decade or more into your practices. However, this does not mean you should not make explorations and dedicate some of your meditative time in this direction. After all, that could be the difference between entering this profound state of existence or being caught in the illusion. Just, remember to do the foundations, such as kriya, moving energy, integration, compassion, communion, life's lessons and eternal yoga.

There is often confusion around the semantics of how the term "central channel" is used within different contexts by various authors. All are valid, provided you understand the context in which it is used. The term central channel can indicate a common energy flowing in the spinal marrow, it can also indicate a profoundly deep energy flowing within the spinal marrow. As this deep energy is beyond the physical body, this same pathway can also be connected with through visualizing a pathway in front of the spinal marrow. As long as you are connecting with a profound core of your being, either of the last two examples are valid for our purposes. When I use the term, central channel it is in relation to the deep pathway of the last two definitions, and not a common electrical energy also running through the spinal marrow. As we become more integrated, however, the central channel also includes this common energy within it. Also as this more common energy is what helps us to firm our attention within the central channel, it is easy to see how this can be called the central channel. Reality is a continuum not dictated to by the needs of authors wanting to create black and white directions.

Other names for the central channel include the fusion channel, the thrusting channel and the amrit nadi. However even here semantics can again vary the meaning. For example, in accord with acupuncture theory and application, the fusion or thrusting channel runs along the spinal marrow, is deeply connected to the kidney energy and runs up the front on two routes, one to each side of the frontal line. There are also additional branches This has a deep energetic resonance and truth to our description of the central channel, even if they appear different. When one is in the central channel, you can feel both the front (frontal line) and back (spinal marrow) of the body emanating from it in a perfect balance, and there is an essence of the kidneys strongly within it (through the water element). Because acupuncture theory is primarily developed for medical reasons, the pathways are related to in relation to healing of the body. This is not always exactly the same as the more mystical uses of the energy flows, which in their deepest realms can take one beyond the body and its appearance of health or disease.

The central channel will only be introduced here, as it is more the subject of the inner tantras (addressed in later books in this series). I do not believe that you can really develop in the fusion channel without a deep connection with and awareness of various highly developed masters. Also, profound development within this channel is concurrent with letting go of self-centered importance into the larger reality of collective existence within the radiant emptiness (what Christians call God), i.e., no longer grasping as the Buddhists say.

It is amazing that so many of the tantras, which of necessity revolve around the central channel use the element of fire to start the blissful increase, absorption and circulation within the channel. It is generally unknown that there are tantras that use the water element instead to do this (I am not talking about sex here). A number of years ago I received a terma (in short, a profound transmission) in this regards (this is the first I have been allowed to mention it), but I need a few more years of application before I can reveal it. At that time a book will be written on it, so for those who are interested, stay tuned.

The central channel is in the center of the body from the genitals up to the top of the head and then to the third eye. It extends above the head and has subtle connections to your roots within the earth. All the other channels spring forth from it, directly or indirectly.

The central channel in relation to the body contains more of a water element than the other channels. For this reason it is often easier for women to intuitively feel it than men.

While firm placement of this channel in the body is absolutely necessary for advanced practice, it is a mistake to think of it as defined by or floating within the body. Rather, it is the other way around. The body (and everything else) comes into being around it. This is how an accomplished master can make their body seemingly disappear, reappear, or change shape.

While the central channel is incredibly sublime, do not make it beyond yourself through mystery, mystique or something that is too advanced. The fusion channel is the "natural" state. It is right within you and can be accessed, and is accessed within many levels of its existence. Thus it is something that you are already working with. It is simply a degree of profound familiarity with and penetration into your own wholesomeness and the feeling that it is all one. Because of its natural way of existence, religious practitioners, even if possessing the yogic skills are sometime too caught up in the contrivance of their path to really enter it, which requires a letting go. From the other camp, those who lack the dharmic disciplines often do not have enough emphasis on the importance of the inner stance and surrender to it to actually remain in and center within the fusion channel. The support offered, service given, shelter received and constant self-reflection in a dharma community is invaluable for a period of time. Thus do your best and in the humility of sincerity keep growing.

Connecting with the central channel is profoundly making love within. This requires a tremendous inner intimacy and willingness to feel consuming passion. It also requires the ability to internalize the energy. Otherwise, while the energy might begin in the proximity of the fusion channel, it will become prematurely dispersed through outer projection, fantasy, or wandering. The central channel greatly assists in being able to work with and absorb cosmic and universal energy.

Being able to fully apply yourself in this consciousness requires a general grounding and purification, a sense of whole-body-feeling, the desire to grow spiritually, a basic compassion for others that has love, the ability to detach when necessary, a somewhat intense and passionate nature, a transparent view of life and the willingness to apply yourself while taking responsibility for that application.

The central channel emanates flows of energy in the body through masculine/feminine pairs. These consist of several sets of subtle flows of energy to the sides of the fusion channel. One of these pairs travels parallel to the fusion channel. Another aspect of this same pair is how it coils around each of the chakras, as an emotional and energetic connection to that chakra. The nature of how this energy coils is not set, but changes. It is similar to how a flow of electricity will curve in to a magnet, yet of a tighter radius. In this case the magnet is love. There is another pair of supporting energy channels about an inch and a half or more to each side of the central channel (this is not the same as the side channels of the outer-spine). This pair coils in a continual helix from bottom to top. It is purely an emotional-energetic expression of the fusion channel. When someone enters the fusion channel through intuitive passion, rather than specific detailed instruction, it is most often through the support of this pair of energy flows. There is distant pair that travels up toward the sides of the torso, connecting to the organs and the belt channel (see following pages). Another primary pair is the microcosmic orbit, consisting of the frontal and spinal channels. The part of the fusion channel between the heart and the head is known as the Amrit Nadi.

Sometimes, dreams of a lucid nature where you watch the sun and moon eclipse are signs of your energy entering into the central channel, although this can also be an indication of your energy entering into the inner earth. In these dreams both the sun and the moon are full. In advanced practice you can dream, where you are totally awake and inside the central channel, and conscious of this channel being inside your sleeping body. Inside this dream, you can travel up and down the channel and have different experiences at different places within it. This is my experience.

As the central channel enters into the head, there are two branches. One goes over the head and down to the third eye, just inside the skull and the other goes to the occipital through the center of the head and to the third eye. It is good to work with both paths, although not necessarily at the same time.

While the microcosmic orbit can be done with the central channel and the frontal channel, as the central channel opens more this is unnecessary as the frontal channel is automatically stimulated just through the resonance effect and outpouring of the central channel. This can be so strong that the frontal channel is actually felt as an integral part of the central channel. However it often occurs that through practice of the microcosmic orbit your energy deepens from the outside of the spine more into the central channel. Also the microcosmic orbit can be split where you feel part of the energy rising up the spine as on the outside of the spine and part of it on the inside of the spine, but again after the energy gets really rich in the central channel, the outer channels are automatically stimulated and included without having to hold any primary focus on them at all. You will know when this happens simply because you will feel it. I feel a good way to circulate energy for the purpose of enlivening the central channel is by using the side channels as it will help to firm up the central channel itself. Also when doing work on the central channel it is good to also do general whole body enlivening exercises.

While it is good to visualize the central channel as large in width at times, even as wide as your body or larger[1], it is better to keep it about the width of your little finger, or even smaller most of the time. Also for many trying to connect with the spinal marrow they actually end up connecting with the outer aspects of the spine instead and thereby generate a mental fire. Thus it can be more helpful to feel the central channel as running up the center of your body. This helps you to get more the proper feeling of it, both in location and as a blending of the frontal and back energy. Later when everything gets more firm, you can nudge it towards the back of the body a bit.

The reason to keep it smaller in size is it aids your penetration and it creates a better atmosphere of emptiness, which is an inherent trait of the central channel. The energy of this mind of emptiness is called Wu chi in Taoist practices and clear light in Tibetan Tantric practices. Do not think that larger, means more energy. This is only true in a very physical sense, and even then you want to create just the right amount of physical energy, not too much, not too little so that the mind is in the right state to achieve the effortless balance. A visualized tube, when softened, deepened and free of blockages the size of your little finger can carry many magnitudes more energy that currently exists in your entire body, so the size is more than sufficient.

The reason to make it bigger at times, is to make it less mentally fixated (i.e., softer) and too help you gain an initial physiological connection with all the energies of your body. Understand that the central channel is not a dull mental energy, it is incredibly alive bliss. You need all of your body's energy focused for some time, repeatedly, to help ignite it, but from there it is a cultivation.

When Mahavatar BabaJi gave the transmission of the Ati of his Body into mine (and a number of other yogis present including Whitecloud), he first absorbed his body into becoming a tube a bit bigger than three inches in diameter, which was the central channel. There was a particular reason for this size, because of particular relationships with cosmic rays, so understand that there are reasons at times the central channel can "appear" bigger or smaller in an advanced yogi, but when you are really in the channel, everything is of it, the dualistic fingers and measures we use to describe it outwardly disappear in non-dual awareness.

1 As is sometimes effectively done in a few eternal yoga visualizations, in some general getting acquainted with the central channel visualizations, and indirectly although very profoundly through the visualizations of (larger) generation stage Tibetan tantras,

ENERGY AND ESSENCES

Energy is also referred to as prana, chi, wind, radiance and life force. The terms are used interchangeably in this book so as to give variety to such a frequent and important word. Understand that various traditions are all built upon verbal and perceptual qualifications of the same underlying principles of natural existence.

Energy is often described by how it has been qualified. This includes elemental characteristics of the earthy, watery, fiery, airy and spatial state. For example, meditating on our deep water qualities, such as in the center of our body and in our bones results in an increase of cool watery refreshing building contained energy. Lots of action, fast thought, and exercise generates a fire quality of energy. Building energy inside of us to hold a focus and then using that focus to open an inner space, develops the space element whereby we can birth new understandings and create energy. By understanding the different qualities of energy needed for physical and spiritual purposes, we can learn how to dynamically generate these energies in the correct balance for our purpose at hand. Examples of what we can achieve with this knowledge is creating a clear mind, creating more life force to accomplish our aims in and enjoyment of life, consuming undesired energy, helping others, and even generating a body of energy-substance that we embody beyond the confines of our present physical time and space.

This language gains incredible value when a practitioner starts to generate and balance the nectars. To those who say, Ha!, we are made of atoms not elemental states, that elemental states are just various degrees of excitement or lack of atoms, such as ice, water and vapor, do not understand the nature of consciousness itself on the primal level of form. The elemental qualities describe feeling states, and it is this feeling sensitivity that IS the bridge (or continuum) from formless consciousness into form.

As consciousness is inseparable from its energy component and in turn the type of consciousness or sensory quality it supports, such as gross, subtle, radiant, particular organ energy; a sense or an emotion may describe energy. Energy is also described by the place it is found such as in the aura, and where it originates from or how it is sensed such as a person, a rock, the astral realm, causal light, and what function or form it takes such as electrical, magnetic, heat, etc.

Essences include various nectars, secretions, and substances of the body, such as blood, semen and hormones. In particular this is in reference to the energetic nature of these substances. Included in this are the subtle nectars found at the center of the chakras and other tangible concentrations of energy.

Essences are the bridge between subtle and physical. Pure essences are held together by (and even made out of) elemental consciousness, i.e., watery, fiery, sublime, and earthy natures in infinite combinations, hues, sounds and subtleties. Essences always have an ecstatic nature. As we ascend (transform our form into consciousness itself) our entire body becomes an essence of our spirit. Tantra is the potency of essences. The spiritual reason to learn about the chakras and channels is the tantric containment, circulation and radiance of our essences.

When our eternally radiant consciousness becomes defined and expanded enough, we begin to live in a core of this essence right within our body. As water is the nature of an ocean so we become aware of our own indivisibility with the ocean of all life, experiencing ourselves through and at times, as the myriad variety within the ocean. The containment and definition of our own essential nature is the means by which we become aware of the nature of our own and every existence. Oneness is first experienced through the oneness of our own self.

Essences are also the bridge between individual and universal consciousness. Individuality is the very means of life itself, without which there is no life. Ingrain this understanding in your practices, that you may feel good about yourself and give yourself the permission to be who you are in your ever-expanding perfection. Individuality, as it becomes refined, remains as an essence that is your presence. What fills the blissful core of your inner temple is your essence-nectar. Individuality is the vehicle or carrier of our universal presence that it may dance in the sea of life. When your presence is experienced as forever emanating in its myriad forms from the emptiness, you have found God.

While our whole body lives in a sea of energy, in applying chi kung and visualization exercises, energy is often first felt as a tingling, like a pleasant current. We can learn how to move energy in this way through connectivity with our mind and/or our breath. For example breathing up the spine and down the sides, while visualizing and sensing a movement of energy, will eventually result in us being able to tangibly feel the energy as it moves along our tissues. We commonly first feel it be the effect it is having on out tissues, but eventually we can learn how to feel energy purely as it self. For example, we can feel an energy current outside our own body, or deep within it beyond physicality.

Learning to create and connect with flows of energy is incredibly valuable for spiritual practices, because we now have the ability to direct our lifeforce into focal points where we can refine and blend the energy into essence. Also with this ability of connectivity, we can learn to circulate and balance our lifeforce.

Of course this refinement and circulation can be done solely through intention and relaxing into a general visualization. For example visualizing ourselves bathing in golden light and everything is perfect. However by relying purely on such a technique it is less likely that we will develop the necessary penetration to progress all the way on the spiritual path. There are vast areas or our emotional-physical-spiritual embodiment we can miss simply miss altogether and it may not occur to us that we even have missed something.

Cultivating nectar substances involves their increase, refinement and containment. Because in our society we have learned that ra ra ra is the way of energy, we may not understand that the best way to create lasting energy in the body is in in in, then ra ra ra. This inward focus when made alive increases refines and contains energy-substance. For example, the sexual organs gain their power through the seminal fluids. These fluids emanate a quality of energy that acts as a template by which the other energy-substance we take into our body such as air, food and environment can emulate. Without this pattern and its wisdom to emulate, new energy we take into the body is raw, somewhat different, unguided and easily scattered. Nectar substances in the body are generators of particular qualities that when they become strong enough dictate the patterns to follow. Without there generators we are always trying to get new energy to become our energy, to behave in a certain way such as making us feel potent or alive or our particular likes. However, with nectar substances, half the work is already done, they are like teachers to all the energy we bring in. They are like batteries that keep on generating particular qualities and this results in stabilization in our meditative insight and thus the vision of what we are flowering into.

Without cultivating nectar and containing it through our spiritualized body, we can have a nice meditation, but an hour later its effects our gone. We can have great sex, but nothing lasts. We can experience enlightenment, but it is fleeting and gone the next moment. However, as our body becomes nectarized, our spirit and body unite, and one remembers the other. Then our meditations build one upon the other, our movements become dance, our efforts bear fruit, and the higher realizations such as buddhic consciousness and the body of oneness (emptiness) come forth easily and as they grow in awareness are maintained without doubt.

Bodily Fluids

Refinement and inward extraction of our blood and seminal fluids into the central channel gives bliss and presence, both essentials aspects of the tantric path.

Seminal fluid binds our creative spirit with form. Seminal fluids, both male and feminine, are easily connected with and thereby can be worked with. As this connectivity is refined, working with seminal fluids begins to enhance an inner radiance. It is this subtle energy component that we control and through which we gain outer control and refinement. It becomes the lifeblood of a subtle body we create right within our physical body.

Semen is not only our immediate sexual fluids, but has an essence component in lymph, bone marrow (including our brains), and a tangible presence in the chakras that can even be excited to the point of orgasmic bliss within those chakras. The primary nature of semen is coolness of a refreshing, present and calm quality that is very connected with the water element.

It is the function of blood to be the carrier of our heat and energy. Blood is both a precursor of and a carrier of seminal essence. Blood is the material that masculine and feminine seminal essence needs to become a physical body. The intimate relationship the navel area has with blood is one of the main reasons this area can so quickly rebalance the health of our body.

Food, breath and movement are the physical components that when properly engaged create clean blood and semen. To inwardly connect to the essence of semen, "feel" it as white and of a sweet, sensual, earthy smell. Seminal fluid is first refined into a kind of oil called Ojas. Thus you can add an oily quality to your meditation of connectivity. Add to this the electrical nature of sexual desire and you have a way of moving this essence in the body.

As Ojas is produced it pervades the entire body, but its principle residence is in the bone marrow including your brain and your kidneys. Becoming aware of your bone marrow is a good way of internalizing your sexual essence so that it becomes strength. While most people would argue that the seat of their sexual fluids is in their genitals, the yogis say that it is in the head. By concentrating on a small white radiance of light at the third eye or in the center of the head, seminal production is increased. Remember that the function of semen is to bind the subtle light into the physical. As the principle entrance of your spirit is through the top of your head, then you may start to understand why the sexual essence is felt to originate in the head. According to the yogis, this very subtle essence descends to the genitals, where it then combines with fluids produced by the body to become semen. By bringing it back up the cycle become complete.

In contrast, the seat of blood is felt to exist in the navel region. While it is true that the heart pumps our blood, the heart does not directly contain or create the qualities of blood. However, in tantric practice, the subtle center of the heart is felt as the perfect blending of semen and blood and infuses both with a spiritual quality. Blood is connected to as a red, warm, slightly oily substance that circulates through the body and receives nourishment from the navel and earth energies.

Kundalini is the movement of essences in the body, essentially the energy of our subtle body within the physical body expressing itself. Thus Kundalini (Kriya) yoga is a practice that integrates our subtle and physical body into a unified expression, thereby revealing the natural state of our beingness.

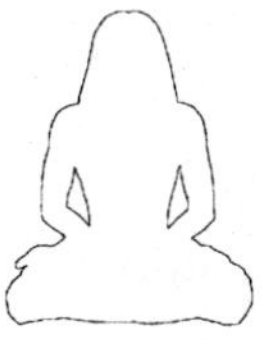

12

Introducing a Tantra of Inner Fire

Vase Breathing, also called kumbhakha, is a method of compressing energy into a small area within the navel area to increase health and to both create our inner temple and center within it. The density of energy created helps to ignite a mystic inner-fire that awakens us into our radiant nature. This fires gathers, stimulates and circulates bliss, which embodied becomes nectar. Nectar sustains us into a 24-hour awareness of our spirit in form, and this is tremendously liberating.

This is not a beginning technique and you should have at least several years of yogic practice under your belt. You should have a cognitive sense of your whole body energy, along with some penetration into the chakras and a reasonably good ability to circulate and transform energy within your body. You should have some experience of what the words body, soul and spirit means more than a vague definition. It is highly recommended that you carefully read the chapter on chakras, channels, energy and essences to compliment this practice.

In the kriyas presented in this book, it is helpful when finishing to inhale and hold the breath for as long as comfortable. As you do so hold the breath deep in the abdomen, pull the navel in, pull up a slight mhula-bhand, keep the neck straight and slightly tensed and keep absorbing the energy into the navel chakra. Then as you exhale, exhale it up in a controlled fashion through the spine and into the head. If done correctly you will feel an exhilarating sense of clearness and grounded lightness. If you hold the energy at the solar plexus rather than below the navel, you will experience burps and may create a bloating in your stomach.

While holding the breath is generally only done once at the end of a kriya, such as a chant or pranayama, vase breathing makes this into a whole technique in itself. As such you practice inhaling, holding the breath, pushing down, pulling up from below, compressing and transforming the energy, then exhaling, repeatedly for 15 minutes to an hour per session. Take some normal breaths whenever you need to. It is important that this is only down by a fit and healthy person without heart complications. If you do have health problems, then practice only with the gentle visualizations as described in the preliminary breathing and visualization section on the next page. Also it is not to be practiced by woman on their moon cycles or while pregnant.

While vase breathing is used in several yogic paths including various Kriya, Taoist and Buddhist lineages, it is perhaps best known as a technique introduced within the completion stage practices of some Tibetan Buddhist tantras such as the Six Yogas of Naropa. It is important to distinguish that vase breathing is not of itself these tantras, which are much more involved than just vase breathing.

Inner fire tantra is a practice, itself used in a variety of different tantric practices, to absorb our energy and attention within the central core of our being in a relationship with our body, particularly through the navel chakra. Once we have obtained sufficient identification with this aspect of ourselves (or as popularly stated, "overcoming ordinary appearances"), then we cultivate nectars which increases the totality and naturalness of these realization through the power of consuming non-dual bliss/wisdom consciousness.

If you are looking to this technique to obtain higher tantric completion stage realizations by igniting the spirit-fire at the navel chakra, then you should understand that in the process of compressing the prana, we are not just creating a heat, but bridging these pranas and sensations into an incredibly deep dimension and continuum of ourselves, and using this process as a way of stabilizing a very refined awareness. While a good introduction is given here, all of the preparations and intricacies of this process are really beyond the scope of any book, and are best learned from a competent teacher over an extended period of instruction and feedback[2]. Thus what is given here, in terms of awakening the blissful inner-fire and using it for spiritual practice, is an introduction. The actual process is as much science as art, and being a science it is not limited to one particular framework, for example the Tibetan form of deity identification to achieve the necessary activations, the particular letter forms used to create a focus and container for subtle energy, etc. But also understand that there is an incredible wisdom and power of lineage transmission in how different systems, such as the Tibetan tantras apply these techniques into a complete application.

The subtle and pleasant heat ignited by inner-fire practices, such as vase breathing, is not composed of just fire, but all the elements in a particular balance. Do not be mislead with the term "fire," for the water element is just as important in this practice, for some even more important. Without understanding this balance, which is slightly different for each of us according to our constitution, difficulty can arise. Our subtle channels must be reasonably clear, and we need a transparent understanding of ourselves. Furthermore, this heat is not an ordinary heat in the body, and finally it is a vehicle that you must learn how to drive to your destination, not the destination itself.

To give an idea of where this heat centered deep in the body is ultimately ignited from (the sambogakaya realm), for myself I have experienced it most strongly through the activation of part of my central channel about four feet above my head, then the reflection into the body effortlessly blazes the inner fire. This is a level of transmission that occurs from the masters, not just visualization. This does not mean you should abandon more conventional body orientated practice, but understand the continuum of what you are opening up into.

For those who have had some yogic experience, and are attracted to do an intense practice involving vase breathing, by all means practice, but also be prepared to seek out further assistance as you advance and questions arise. For those who just want to be more centered and gain health benefits, then practice in proportion to that desire. As long as you listen to what your body is saying, then you have a built in check and balance system. Do not be scarred away by an image of complexity, but also respect what is said and keep a perspective.

Preliminary Breathing and Visualizations

It is helpful to do some warm-up stretching and movement to open us up a bit. Then sit comfortable with a straight spine, create a space of blessings for your practice and dedicate this blessing. If you are pressed for time, it is permissible to make this blessing initiation of your practice short, otherwise take the time to really connect with and feel this blessing presence for you, and from you. It makes the difference. Without developing connectivity to a blessing presence, your practice will always remain on an outer level. While yogic techniques are all quite scientific, the universe is consciousness and it is the blessings of higher consciousness beings that reveal its ultimate penetrating secrets of unbound love and light.

Now visualize the spinal marrow. Feel it as inwards, in fact when you connect to the cool intimate presence of your spinal marrow it will feel more towards the center of your body as if your spine was behind it.

Breathe up and down one side of the spine for a few minutes, then repeat on the other side. You do not need to block one of your nostrils with a finger, simply visualize the breath going down the side of the spine and back up it. There are multiple routes of energy that run parallel to the spine. The ones further out are more connected to denser emotions, and the flows closer to the spine are connected to a refined emotional sense of oneself. Until we refine our emotions, it is difficult to get our energy to want to stay close to the spine in this practice.

For the next breathing preliminary, as you inhale, feel that you are inhaling the breath up the spine starting from the tailbone all the way up the spine to the top of the head and then down to the forehead and when you are finished inhaling pause at the third eye area holding the breath for a few moments. As you inhale, make sure that your physical breath is going down into your navel area, even though your subtle breath is moving up the spine, otherwise you may experience chest pains. Then exhale in a very focused manner down one side of the spine keeping the energy as close to the spine as possible. As you finish the breath pause for a few moments at the tailbone while holding the breath out and absorb the prana at that point. Repeat a dozen times on one side, and then the same for the other side. As your energy starts to circulate into the tailbone it will make you feel light, at ease, transformative and joyful. As you gather energy in the forehead, it will open a wonderful inner sense, help to dissolve the residue of too much thinking and increase your ability to focus. Be sure to visualize that your breath is composed of an energy substance. After a month or two of practice you will actually feel this tangible enjoyable energy-substance.

These preliminaries will help immensely. In fact there are wonderful practices in particular kriya lineages where something similar to this is done for hours, with the added benefit that the presence and image of particular masters are held within the prana being circulated and at various points. Because of the particular transmissions of these masters, and some other fine points, this fuller version may only be given through private initiation to those who are ready. But the basic version described above will still be of great assistance for the purposes presented here.

By concentrating energy close to the spine, we help to firm the energy path of the spine itself. Commonly when people visualize their spine, they will be directing their attention on the outer part. This results in a mental fiery energy and is not what is used for this practice, rather we need to get inwards into the marrow. When this is done, our awareness and energy flowing through the spine will be more refreshing, cool and ecstatic in nature. As we open into the deep qualities of the spine, we enter more into the central channel, also known as the fusion channel. This will feel quite deep in the body, more towards its center and have a resonance with both our back and front. It is not located in our physical body, so understand that various types of practice will describe different ways of anchoring it into a relationship with the physical. There are a number of vertical energy pathways on each side of the spine, and by bringing the energy close into the spine, really close, we help to shift from what is called the governing channel to the correct aspect of the central channel that is used for this practice. Also by breathing and visualizing energy into the side channels, we heal and energize our bodies energy and can thereby bring it into a relationship within the central channel through one of its chakras.

Now penetrate to find that place an inch or two below the navel and more towards your back than the front. For those of you familiar with Taoist practices, this is not the dan tien nor is it the ming men point (on the governing channel), actually it is central to them both. You will know it when you find it. Visualize yourself as a small warm extremely radiant red presence within that place. Remember that you are firming your energy in the abdominal area to help hold a place of sustained focus within it, but that the actual point is not in the physical. However energy can both move into it from and out to the physical from it. Your outer body develops a relationship to it. Do not be disheartened if it takes many months to get everything roughly in place, this is actually more the norm. The smaller you can make the point of light, the more easier it is to enliven it as pure spirit, but the more difficult it is to initially ground within the bodies physiological support mechanism and thus harder to maintain continuously. The larger it is, the easier it is too connect it with all of our emotional and physiological presence, but it becomes more bound to our conventional existence and thus for most of us, less (effortlessly) bright. Eventually we learn how to make a very small point of pure spirit that has many layers of radiant clothing known as our body and all its feelings. Thus a continuum is established.

As discussed in the chapter on chakras and channels, we can visualize our central channel from being the width of our body (or wider) to a thin tube. There are various outer aspects and inner aspects of the central channel. The difference is that the outer aspects, while having a magnetic blissful and absorption/radiance quality, lacks the fullness of our true nature as radiant emptiness. Unless we have already established ourselves in emptiness understanding, then we will not do so in these outer aspects. By making the central channel small in diameter, and when we can absorb our pranas into it, we will automatically be in an atmosphere to correctly understand emptiness. It is in this atmosphere that we can truly transform, purify ourselves and understand our true nature. For example, in the understanding of emptiness you could visualize a pile of excrement and instantly transform it into an honest experience of perfume and nectar, however in regular visualization most likely we would be grossed out, at least I would. This understanding of emptiness, or radiant presence, is not something we should force or try to grasp at, rather it just becomes more apparent within us (over years of practice). This is what enlightenment is, and through enlightenment we can apply ourselves into greater enlightenment.

Another benefit of using visualization along with directing the breath with the mind in its correct course, is that this will help to awaken the visual ability within these very refined pranas. This is not forced, it is not imagination, we are not trying to imagine seeing anything, rather it is the connectivity of grounding, of definition, of awareness. Thus it is important that in our visualization of the breath along the spine, of our bright red presence, and of all the creative tools we use, we gain the ability to be able to steadily apply a visual sense without forcing, blinding, or distorting it through expectation and ambition.

From within this radiant aspect of ourselves, feel a rich magnetic quality that all on its own attracts the pranas of your body and environment into us as this small red light. From below, feel our sensual, potent, sexuality arise and join into our focus. In fact, just this visualization if practiced consistently enough will ignite the inner fire without vase breathing at all. However for most of us our minds tend to wander, our energy is not vital enough and we need a little extra physical help, and this is the purpose of vase breathing, to provide that help.

Vase Breathing

The length of practice depends on the individual. Gently inhale a full breath, swallow a small amount of saliva and press the breath down to the navel area. Pull your energy up from your anus and genitals, slightly pull the stomach in, and press everything together at a point an inch or two below the navel and more towards the back than the front. You want it to be pulled in by and guided to the small bright red presence of yourself in the navel chakra. This is similar to using a bellows to fan a fire. The reason it is called vase breathing is that the breath is held, like in a vase, compressed from above and below.

Hold for as long as comfortable, and then release the breath into this point and up the spine into the head. However, do not release all the energy too quickly upwards. If you do then all that energy may rush up on the outside of the spine, or up some other way and cause you to feel dizzy. If you do get dizzy, stop and regain your composure. If you understand how to meditatively pull the energy back into the channels then do so, otherwise do some stretches and then meditate to bring your mind back into a clear focus. Then continue, but carefully. Common causes of dizziness are pushing yourself too quickly in the beginning, tiredness (do not practice when tired), and/or the mind wandering. If your mind is wandering bring it under control **before** you start vase breathing. You want the energy to become absorbed into the navel chakra and in the process transform itself into a finer substance. Thus I found it helpful, at first, to keep the energy at the navel while exhaling, rather than allowing it to burst upwards. After awhile the prana gets more condensed at the navel, and will start to want to move upwards in the intimate atmosphere of the inner channel, and without dizziness. As an analogy, it is similar to trying to direct high-pressure air, which wants to go any which way it can. As the gas is condensed into a liquid, the liquid can be contained easier and directed. It is much easier to control in this way, and one of the primary purposes of vase breathing is learning to control our energy.

For those with aspirations to ignite the true inner-fire of bliss, if you do not learn how to control the energy at this level, then it will be impossible to channel your energy as its gets stronger and your conventional sense of self changes. As another analogy, think of the difficulty in holding back, or even wanting to, an impending orgasm in sexual climax and you will begin to understand what is meant by this.

If you try to force vase breathing too much, you may start to become more angry, fanatical, and sharp with people. The water element will be missing, and while you think you are being a yogi, you will in fact only become a pain to others. These are all signs that the fire element is moving out of balance. Soften up a bit in your practice and take your time. Trying to create an inner heat without the support of water will only burn you up. It is not so much inner heat we want, rather inner intimacy and this involves softness and a very alive seductive quality of absorption.

Remember that I mentioned in the beginning of these instructions, that what is presented here is not a full set of instructions. Some people can read between the lines, can apply the other aspects of what they know through years of practice, and reap a lot. This is not because I want to hold anything back from you; rather the entirety of our spiritual evolution simply cannot be presented in one technique. If you are expecting certain results, and they are not forthcoming, it may be because there are other areas of your being that needs development. For example, your may need a conscious transmission and follow through with practice of what your innermost nature is like. You may need to meditate on what the nature of radiant emptiness is, or you may need to loosen up your self-importance to experience what your inner nature is. You may need more practice with visualization or learning how to feel your subtle breath (practice the microcosmic orbit presented later in the book). There may be emotional healing that need precedence. There may simply be an appropriateness of timing and grace, or there may be some physical correction of technique. Or your path may be entirely different and for you that path is more effective. Finally you may just need more patience. It is important to have confidence in your practice, and that is what a qualified teacher can help your with.

Do not hold the breath in extreme discomfort, or force this technique. What will likely happen if you do, is that you will be emphasizing the physical aspect of it too much and the energy will remain on an outer level. You may create heat flushes or flashes in the body, which is also an indication that the energy is remaining outward. The correct heat, when it eventually comes is a small very deep thick heat that stays put and can gradually be expanded and circulated. It is not so much the heat that is important, rather the indescribable delicate non-dual feeling quality of bliss that is invoked, the heat is just a product of the prana being so activated, although it is inseparable from the experience. In fact there are other tantric means, less well known, that do not even start with heat, but some other elemental quality. Do not be in a rush. Sometimes you simply ignore the breath altogether and hold presence at the prescribed point within the navel chakra and magnetically pull your bodies energy into that place through seduction. This is also a recommended way to end your vase breathing session.

You have to coordinate growth in this practice with ability through your being as a whole, subtly, emotionally and spiritually. For example, many people when they first start meditating at the third eye experience a wandering of mind, or if they hold the energy well headaches and eyeaches. The subtle channels need to become clear, the dross of intellectual thought washed away and the nectar that can hold this energy increased. Then it is effortless, but this takes time and consistency with a gentle focus. Thus when you start bringing up extra energy into the head, you will feel it in your occipitals, all over your head and in your forehead. As you build up the nectars, then their is the proper container. Also as you develop a whole body feeling, then energy circulates through the whole body.

In the first few weeks, as you inhale you simply bring the energy down, and press it down while pulling up, trying to find the exact point at the navel chakra. After these first few weeks, feel that you are inhaling the breath simultaneously down both sides of the spine and as you push down, you are squeezing the breath down the two sides of the spine. These energy routes along the spine become very full and charged with energy, and thus these is really something there to mix into the center. This makes it much easier to direct it into the navel center.

If this is too difficult, then spend more time in the preliminary visualization and breathing. Also try the following technique. Breathe normally and feel your whole abdominal area increase with energy as you breath. Feel a point near the surface of your skin, in all four directions, i.e., at your tan-tien, at your spine, at each side. As you continue to breath, gently feel this energy spiraling into the center. Feel that you are sitting and practicing in a large vibrant field of alive-energy within and around you, blessed with many sacred beings, and continue to absorb it all into the bright red presence in the center. This does not have to be only red in color. Sometimes an orange can give it more of a fluid sensual bliss, white can give it combinations of earth, moisture, and subtly depending in how it is felt, gold or yellow can increase confidence and substance; experiment, but it is recommended to mainly stay with a blood red.

In the beginning months of practice, you may have gas and your abdomen may get bloated at times. This is all simply purification, clearing of blockages and muscle weakness. It can also result form stagnation of energy, because you are creating energy in one area, holding it there, but not transforming it. Remember the golden rule, unless you are under expert instruction, back off on your length of practice when necessary and proceed gradually. Then everything will have time to adjust and you will have the time to mature into it. Also, anyone doing this practice should also be doing other forms of meditation as part of their overall practice. This is a must. For example, contemplation on or with spiritual beings, deep meditation, kriya or chi kung practice, exercise, etc.

There are several excellent complimentary practices. One of these is martial arts horse stance. In the stance, sit deeply, and as the stance starts to get a bit intense, feel yourself pushing the energy down into the navel and pulling it up from below. This will give you the correct feeling of mixing the energy. You can also do some short holdings of the breath as you do the mixing. Because of all the energy you are generating from your legs and bringing up from the earth, this really is a great way to learn how to mix energy in vase breathing. When I teach vase breathing, I also teach horse stance with it.

Learning and practicing the microcosmic orbit as outlined later in this book will help keep everything in balance. Before beginning a serious practice of vase breathing you should already be at ease with the microcosmic orbit. Then vase breathing will increase the energy available for its circulation. Also understand that an intense practice of vase breathing and the meditation which follows in its after effect is designed to bring the energy into the central (fusion) channel which is more primal than the microcosmic orbit.

Another excellent complimentary practice is various ways of dissolving normal awareness of your body altogether. For example, set yourself in a meditative posture and feel a blessing presence above your head. Then feel everything around you as light and yourself as light. Feel all of this being seductively absorbed, vanishing into a point inside of yourself, such as at your navel, your heart or throat. Rest in the sense of inner space.

Or do the transparent body practice, where you feel your skin as light-substance, and everything inside as calm empty space with a tinge of white light. Stay with it for awhile, to honestly get into the experience of it. It is amazing and also acts as a training in itself to acclimize you towards more subtle experience. This helps to balance your energy, which is important if you create an imbalance through forcing the energy too much in vase breathing. In addition to dissolving blockages, transparent body practice helps to take all that energy you have created and transform it into finer and finer levels of energy that can circulate and enter into your innermost spaces in perfect balance. All your problems, at least for the moment, elegantly vanish into pure space which is so beautiful.

Another age-old way of balancing our energy is drinking a glass of water and taking a nap.

As our red warm radiance grows stronger, it entices a response in the body. Our sexual desire increases. Our confidence increases. Our spiritual wonder increases; everything increases. It is important that we do not abandon ourselves to the winds, but maintain a sense of control, containment and direction. Once we gain enough internal definition to stay awake in our subtlety, we practice dissolving all of increased sense of self into formless form, and then bring it all back again into ordinariness, again and again and again. If we not dissolve and reform ourselves again and again, then we will mislead ourselves in our seeming importance and in this grasping we will sabotage the real possibility of what our practice can reveal to us. We practice bringing our warm nectar light up the body and back down again, slowly, slowly and consciously, a few inches at a time, pausing and exploring along the way. This is very refreshing. We awaken totally free of constrictions, rules, yet ever aware that we do not exist independent of anything, and thus responsible to everyone in our light of love.

As you may have picked up by now, vase breathing is only to help this ignition, the real mediation is in the aftereffect.

Practice Times and Schedule

You may notice that I do not say 3 or 5 or 10 or 36 repetitions, or practice for 31 minutes, etc. It is important that you do what is right for you, and make sure that in the first weeks it is a little less than you think you can do. For those who need a start, here is a general example for practice. This is primarily for those who want to get into the practice.

For those who just want to practice vase breathing, without all the visualizations as a health benefit to improve their health, then 5 or 10 minutes at a time when you feel like it is a good yardstick, being careful to hold the breath for only a moderate time, and not when you are really tired or your mind is scattered.

If you are not interested in transforming your sensual energy into spiritual bliss and presence, then it is not time for you to do this practice, straight forward and simple with no argument. For a man, this means that he must be willing to do his best to contain his semen. If the ability is not present to hold semen in sex, then it is advisable to be celibate when practicing inner-fire practice. You need your energy strong and contained.

- Do just the preliminary visualizations and breathing for a month. Also do other types of practice such as kriyas, chi kung, dynamic yoga sets, etc. These can be during the same session or at another time.

- Then add on vase breathing for 5 or 10 minutes for a few weeks. For most people they may hold the breath for about 30 seconds and take some long deep relaxed breaths in between. Over time, gradually increase to about a half hour to 40 minutes of vase breathing with none or occasional relaxing breaths inbetween.

- Then follow with 15 minutes to an hour of continuing the generation and absorption of energy just with subtle meditation alone. Finally a heart felt prayer of dedication for the benefit of others concludes the practice session.

- This is all done on an empty stomach. Practicing everyday is best and early morning is a good time. If you do not practice everyday, then every other day. If you practice in the evening and you have had a long day at work and are tired, then warm up with another kind of practice, if your energy does not shift, then do not include the physical part of the vase breathing, because trying to generate, compress, and direct large amounts of physical prana when you are tired is not a good idea. If you cannot control the energy no benefits are gained, and you can do yourself temporary harm.

Variations

There are a number of movements you can do while holding your breath in vase breathing, that help to make you more limber and further clear various channels in the body. The simplest is to place you hands on your knees, and rotate your body from the waist a number of times one direction and then a number of times the other. Another is to do the above and finish by flexing your spine forward and backwards.

As you get better at holding the energy at the specific spot, you will begin to feel effortlessness and that your body is an outer show of your inner self. Instead of being on the outside looking in, you are on the inside radiating out. After you fist begin to feel this, you may want to try the following exercises:

While holding your breath, wriggle and shake your whole body, quickly. Move your hands over your head at times, and really move. Another technique is while holding the breath, to place you fists on the ground besides you and lift your body up and down rapidly, while never loosing that inner place in the navel.

As you increase the inner fire, then practice moving it up and down the central channel, while keeping a connectivity to the its seat in the navel chakra. This will dramatically increase the nectar within your whole being. As this fire (and our general practices) refines our sexual fluids and transports them into the head, and as the nectar spaces in out head become full, then a sweetness drips back down into the body. You may first experience it as a honey-like quality in your saliva. Your goal is to gently excite the nectars in your head. Notice I use the word gently, because control must be present every step of the way. These nectars are very sensual and thus have a direct stimulation of your genitals. When the nectars start flowing down from the head, it is vitally important that you maintain a connection to the spiritual dimension within head centers, often maintained through the third eye or sometimes through a type of breath at the crown center. This also creates a kind of emotional detachment from the desire body. For those who do not yet have the understanding of this type of dynamic within this type of practice, then do not intellectualize about attachment, detachment, desire, etc., within the experiential application of this practice you will understand.

If you try to whip up the fires and melt the nectars to experience lots of bliss, without control, then it will get away from you. As a man, you will most likely have wet dreams, or even some emissions during your practice. The body will not be able to hold the energy and it will try to balance itself through emission. This will hinder your practice. For a woman, you will create uncomfortableness for yourself and topsy-turvy emotions. You may create subtle forces of hinderance.

In the process this helps to give definition to your central channel. As this builds you will feel yourself as a spiritual being 24 hours a day. It is a presence inside, very natural, non-grasping, unforced and radiant. Everything of yourself that is not of this frequency will be consumed by and integrated by it or else these less-enlightened aspects of yourself will try to assert their importance and become a resistance to practice, so this is an educational and healing process that takes time. Be both kind and vigilant with yourself. Learn to contain and cultivate the energy in each chakra. You are creating a body of nectar.

Sometimes, instead of mixing the energy at the navel you will do so at the base of the spine. Sometimes you may build up some energy on your frontal line, not by holding the breath, but simply through visualization and a feeling of vital fullness. The frontal line is a projection of and storage of our emotional nourishing aspect, and this should be full and healthy. Then our practice is natural and more likely to be successful. As you may begin to see, there are a lot of aspects to this practice, and we have only touched on some of them here. However enough has been given to start and carry you forward to your next step. While there may seem to be a lot, it is actually all very simple, exceedingly so when it all comes together. The bliss simply is and while nothing needs to be understood in this bliss, everything is.

Appendix

Contact Info, Web Site, Books

Contact Details:

Virochana Khalsa
PO Box 747
Crestone, CO 81131
mvk@silverearth.com *you can also send an email from our web site*

Books of Light Publishing
PO Box 576
Crestone, CO 81131

Our Web Site:

www.sacredmountainretreat.org

includes

Teaching schedule
About Sacred Mountain Retreat Center
Personal retreats
Articles and information of interest.
Extracts and reviews of books and videos
(which are for sale at a discount price on the site)
Tonic herbal formulas by Sacred Mountain Herbs

This dynamic site is continually being updated and added to.
Our Books are also available on www.crestonemall.com

Additional Books and Videos *from Books of Light Publishing :*

In addition to the following books, we have a number of videos planned, including one currently in production. Stay tuned through our web site for further information.

Tantra of the Beloved

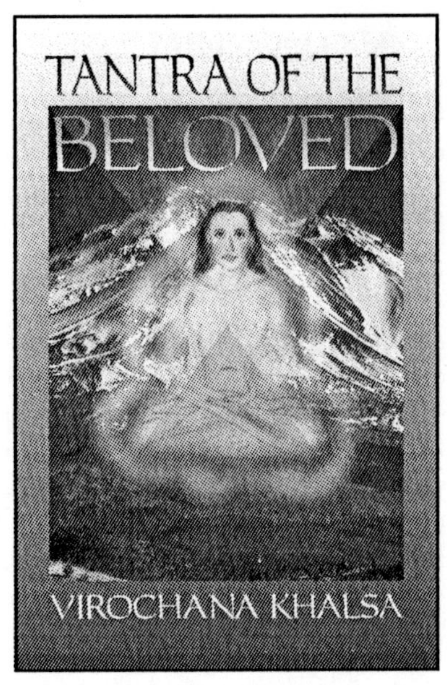

by Virochana Khalsa
ISBN 0-9598048-9-7
600 pages $21.95

Finding Fulfillment in Life, Tantra, Emotions, Awakening a Body of Light, The Empowered Man and Woman, The Beloved Twin Ray, The Ascended Masters, Stellar Karmas, The Inner Earth and More...

The Way of the Goddess, A Journey of Self Awakening

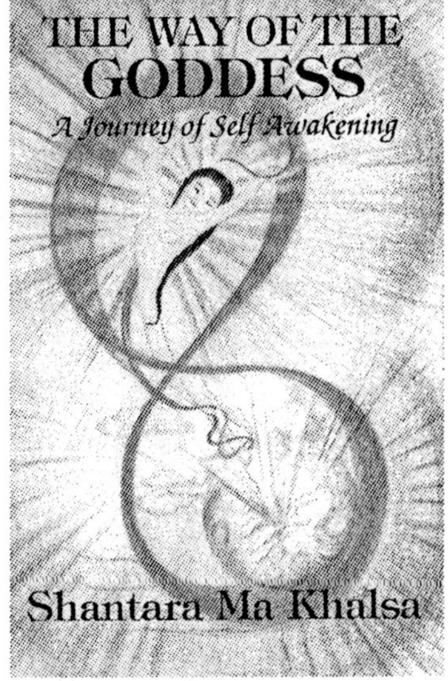

By Shantara Ma Khalsa
(aka Whitecloud)
ISBN 9598048-3-8
224 pages $11.95

An exciting, easy to read and transformational biography of her trials, difficulties and victories in her spiritual path and the quest to meet her beloved. Selected by the New Zealand International Woman's Book Festival.

Tantra Unveiled, through the feminine

by Whitecloud Khalsa
ISBN 1-929952-03-1
144 pages $14.95

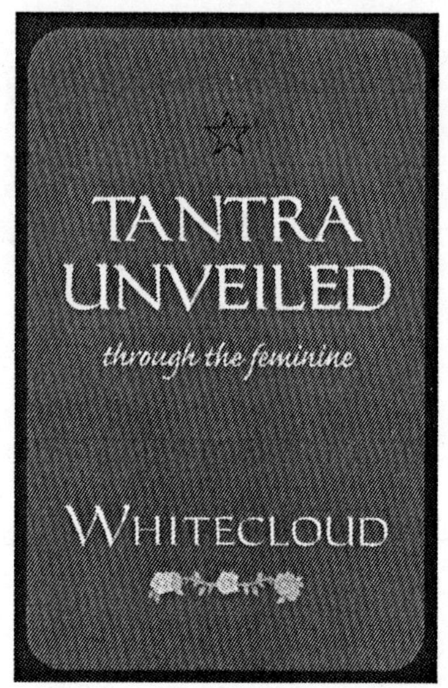

Tantra is a sacred doorway to the secret teachings, opened by mystics who embrace Divine Union.

The revelations and wisdom imparted in this book are from an experienced yogini. Whitecloud received the essence of Tantra from her first Master in India as a young woman, and has further developed this path with the assistance of numerous ascended Masters and her Twin-Ray.

This book is invaluable for anyone wanting to know the totality of what Tantra is as a spiritual path.

Coming Soon

Eternal Yoga, Awakening into Buddhic Consciousness

by Virochana Khalsa
ISBN 1-929952-05-8 $21.95

Creating an Eternal Body through the Higher Tantras

(title may change)

by Virochana Khalsa

9 781929 952045